STUDENT PRACTICE SUPERVISION & ASSESSMENT

A GUIDE FOR NMC NURSES & MIDWIVES

JO LIDSTER
SUSAN WAKEFIELD

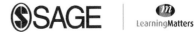

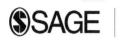

Learning Matters
An imprint of SAGE Publications Ltd
1 Oliver's Yard
55 City Road
London EC1Y 1SP

SAGE Publications Inc.
2455 Teller Road
Thousand Oaks, California 91320

SAGE Publications India Pvt Ltd

B 1/I 1 Mohan Cooperative Industrial Area
Mathura Road
New Delhi 110 044

SAGE Publications Asia-Pacific Pte Ltd
3 Church Street
#10-04 Samsung Hub
Singapore 049483

Editor: Donna Goddard
Development editor: Eleanor Rivers
Senior project editor: Chris Marke
Project management: Swales & Willis Ltd, Exeter, Devon
Marketing manager: Tamara Navaratnam
Cover design: Wendy Scott
Typeset by: C&M Digitals (P) Ltd, Chennai, India
Printed in the UK

Library of Congress Control Number: 2018957325

British Library Cataloguing in Publication data

A catalogue record for this book is available from the British Library

ISBN 978-1-4739-6328-3
ISBN 978-1-4739-6329-0 (pbk)

At SAGE we take sustainability seriously. Most of our products are printed in the UK using responsibly sourced papers and boards. When we print overseas we ensure sustainable papers are used as measured by the PREPS grading system. We undertake an annual audit to monitor our sustainability.

Contents

About the authors

Dr Jo Lidster is a Principal Lecturer in the Department of Nursing and Midwifery at Sheffield Hallam University. Jo leads on learning, teaching and assessment developments for the department as well as supporting placement learning initiatives. She has had a number of key roles including leading research and innovation and research informed teaching developments as well as course leader roles. Jo is an adult nurse and prior to working in education worked in and managed acute and critical care settings. She teaches a range of undergraduate and postgraduate courses in the areas of research methods and evidence-based practice, healthcare education and supporting learners in practice. Jo's research interests include supporting practice areas with new ways of working.

Susan Wakefield is the Deputy Head of Nursing and Midwifery at Sheffield Hallam University. She is responsible for the department's postgraduate and international portfolio. This includes working closely with stakeholders and practice partners to develop a quality learning experience. During her time in higher education, Susan has worked at department, faculty and university level in a number of roles. She is a mental health nurse and had a range of roles in clinical practice including research nurse, care pathways coordinator and community mental health nurse. She teaches research methods and evidence-based practice and supervises postgraduate students.

About this book

This book is a handbook; an easy-to-use guide for Nursing and Midwifery Council (NMC) registrants who are involved in supervising and assessing nursing and midwifery students in practice settings. You may be a newly qualified nurse or midwife or possibly have a wealth of experience in supervising and assessing students. You may be at the start of your supervisor journey or you may have already completed an NMC-approved mentor preparation programme. Either way, we think you will find this book useful. For those of you with less experience of supervising students, it includes information and activities to enhance your understanding of supervising in practice. This includes educational theories and evidence-based models to develop your supervisor attributes and skills. For the reader who is more experienced in student supervision, the book clearly describes the new NMC standards and roles, and suggests how these can be applied to your practice. We intend that it also stretches your understanding and enhances your practice regardless of your existing knowledge and experience. As a result, we hope the book enables you to provide the best learning experience for students, while protecting the public through robust assessment processes.

It is not intended that you read the book from start to finish, or necessarily cover to cover. However, we suggest you do start with Chapter 1, which is an introduction and then *dip into* the rest of the book as you see fit. If you are new to supervising students, you may wish to read each chapter in order. If you are an established supervisor or assessor, you may find it more helpful to focus on specific sections or chapters. The contents page and chapter aims at the beginning of each chapter will help you choose which are most relevant to you.

The book is closely mapped to the new NMC *Standards Framework for Nursing and Midwifery Education* published in 2018. These standards have replaced the NMC *Standards to Support Learning and Assessment in Practice* (2008). This book aims to bring the standards to life and help you apply them in your professional practice. We have mapped the content from each chapter against *Part 1: Standards Framework for Nursing and Midwifery Education* (NMC, 2018d) so you can clearly identify how the chapters relate to these. We have also mapped each chapter's content to relevant professional standards from the Code (NMC, 2015). We have done this to help you recognise how the two are interlinked, as well as to support your NMC revalidation where you are required to map your learning against the Code.

Why this book?

We intend the book to be used as a handbook, containing the most important information about student supervision and assessment in a straightforward and accessible way. We hope you find this easy to refer to and helpful to you in your role as a practice supervisor and/or assessor.

It is not designed to be a theoretical book focusing on the evidence base for educational approaches. However, we do refer to educational and interpersonal theories and models where relevant. We use these for you to consider how they might help you understand your role and develop your attributes and skills. It is a highly applied book, and we have referred to relevant theories and evidence in a way that compliments the NMC standards. There are a number of scenarios and activities; these are included to develop your knowledge and skills as well as help you to apply the standards. We hope you view this book as a critical friend – something you can refer to and receive guidance from to boost your skills and confidence.

Book structure

The book is largely structured around the NMC *Standards for Student Supervision and Assessment* (2018). The chapter titles of Chapters 2–6 directly reflect the sections of these standards. The additional chapters complement the standards and add some further perspectives to supervising and assessing students.

Chapter 1: Introduction to supervision and assessment in practice. This chapter describes the new standards and what the responsibilities are of those undertaking the new roles. It provides a brief overview of the previous standards as the terms used in these will be something you will encounter on a regular basis. We explore the importance of reflective practice in developing as a supervisor and assessor, as well as for your NMC revalidation. We then look at the wider team who are involved in supporting students and student learning, and how these roles interface. We also introduce new and emerging models for organising student support in practice.

Chapter 2: Learning culture. This chapter aims to help you to understand the best learning environment for students to thrive in and be able to meet all the requirements of their placement and educational programme. After reading the chapter and completing the activities, you should have a better understanding of features of a good learning environment. It will help you develop your understanding of not only your role in developing a great learning culture but the role of colleagues and partners in making this happen. We also consider how to support students with diverse needs and those who may have learning contracts and require reasonable adjustments.

Chapter 3: Educational governance and quality. The governance and quality processes that need to be implemented to ensure safe and effective delivery of student learning and assessment are covered in this chapter. These processes and decisions need to be robust to protect the public. We include which processes need to be in place to recruit students onto programmes and ensure safe practice learning environments. We also describe the governance involved in supporting students who are struggling or indeed those who fail to achieve their placement learning outcomes. There is a section on students' *fitness to practise* issues and how to manage this. Finally, we consider how to support students who escalate concerns about poor practice which they have observed while on placement.

Chapter 4: Student empowerment. This chapter summarises the evidence base in relation to how people learn, including learning theories and styles. Understanding how we learn can empower us to take control of our own learning requirements and become self-directed. We suggest how you might adapt your teaching and learning approaches to accommodate different learning styles and preferences thereby creating the best environment for a range of students. The chapter then considers other learning and teaching approaches you can adopt such as peer learning and interprofessional learning. We conclude with examining how generational differences may impact on learning and how you, as supervisor and/or assessor, can facilitate learning opportunities that will appeal to a range of generations.

Chapter 5: Supervisors, assessors and educators. The skills and attributes required of supervisors and assessors and how you can develop these are the focus of this chapter. We also introduce the benefits that can be gained by working collaboratively to support student practice learning. Using learning objectives to maximise learning opportunities is examined, with an aim of supporting your students to be able to recognise their own learning needs. We then outline common teaching methods that you can use in your role and the advantages and disadvantages of these methods. This will provide you with a repertoire of teaching methods to draw upon to meet our students' learning needs wherever possible.

Chapter 6: Curricula and assessment. This chapter will help you recognise your role in understanding and engaging with your student's curricula and develop your understanding of assessment and competence. Understanding assessment approaches and assessment theory is essential in helping us to make robust decisions. We will help you to develop your understanding of different methods that can be used to assess student competence and the benefits of using assessment approaches which involve a range of colleagues. We then examine the importance of feedback including its purpose, benefits of high-quality feedback on learning, and the principles of good feedback.

Chapter 7: Students in difficulty. This chapter builds on earlier chapters where we have introduced students who, for whatever reason, are struggling to progress. We start with examining the term *in difficulty* and the reasons students might find themselves in this position. We help you to more easily identify signs of stress in students and consider the effect it may have on their practice. The chapter includes a model, which can be applied to better support students who are in difficulty. We then move on to assessments and consider how you use processes to manage failing students. Finally we look at how you can look after yourself when supporting the failing student.

Chapter 8: Developing yourself as a supervisor and/or assessor. The focus of this chapter is on you and your developing role as a supervisor and/or assessor. We begin by looking at developing your wellbeing and resilience and the importance of these in your role. We then look at some common and useful techniques for you to develop both your own and your students' resilience. Building on earlier chapters, we consider how useful resilience is when you are working with students in difficulty or when things *go wrong*. The final section of the chapter offers you the opportunity to review your continuing professional development needs. We also suggest how to use your newly acquired knowledge and skills to further develop both your colleagues and your profession.

Learning features

Learning from reading text is not always easy. Therefore, to provide variety and to assist in applying the learning and NMC standards to practice this book contains activities, case studies, scenarios, further reading, useful websites and other materials to enable you to participate in your own learning. You will need to develop your own study skills and *learn how to learn* to get the best from the material. The book cannot provide all the answers – but instead provides a framework for your learning.

Some activities ask you to reflect on aspects of practice, or your experience of it, or the people or situations you encounter. *Reflection* is an essential skill in nursing and midwifery, and it helps you to understand the world around you and often to identify how things might improve. Other activities will help you develop key skills such as your ability to *think critically* about a topic in order to challenge perceived wisdom, and to be able to *make decisions* using that evidence in situations that are often difficult and time-pressured. Communication and working as part of a team are core to all nursing and midwifery practice, and some activities will ask you to carry out *team work activities*. Finally, as a registered nurse or midwife you will be expected to *lead and manage*, and so some activities focus on helping you build confidence in doing this.

All the activities require you to take a break from reading the text, think through the issues presented and carry out some independent study, possibly using the internet. Where appropriate, there are sample answers presented at the end of each chapter, and these will help you to understand more fully your own reflections and independent study.

You might want to think about completing these activities as part of your NMC revalidation. After completing the activity write it up using the NMC revalidation forms and templates (**http://revalidation.nmc.org.uk/welcome-to-revalidation**) and keep it safe so you can use it when it is time for you to revalidate.

This book also contains a glossary on page 159 to assist you with unfamiliar terms. Glossary terms are in bold in the first instance that they appear.

We do hope you enjoy this book and that it helps you on your exciting journey as a supervisor and/or assessor!

Chapter 1   Introduction to supervision and assessment in practice

Standards Framework for Nursing and Midwifery Education. Part 1 of Realising Professionalism: Standards for Education and Training (NMC, 2018d)

This chapter will address all of the standards: **1: Learning culture, 2: Educational governance and quality, 3: Student empowerment, 4: Educators and assessors and 5: Curricula and assessment.**

The Code: Professional Standards of Practice and Behaviour for Nurses and Midwives (NMC, 2015)

This chapter most closely aligns with the following professional standards.

Practise effectively

6.1 make sure that any information or advice given is evidence-based, including information relating to using any healthcare products or services.

6.2 maintain the knowledge and skills you need for safe and effective practice.

  8 work cooperatively (8.1–8.7).

  9 share your skills, knowledge and experience for the benefit of people receiving care and your colleagues (9.1–9.4).

Promote professionalism and trust

20 uphold the reputation of your profession at all times (20.1–20.10).

25.2 support any staff you may be responsible for to follow the Code at all times. They must have the knowledge, skills and competence for safe practice; and understand how to raise any concerns linked to any circumstances where the Code has, or could be, broken.

Chapter aims

After reading this chapter you will be able to:

- describe the key principles of the *NMC Standards for Student Supervision and Assessment*;
- describe the benefits of reflective practice to your role as supervisor/assessor;
- understand the roles of team members involved in supporting learners in practice;
- understand some models used to support learners in practice.

Introduction

Think back to when you were a student. Remember how you felt on those first few hours or days in a new placement area. What helped to settle your nerves and develop your confidence? For many of us it was a mentor or supervisor: the person who welcomed us into their world and guided us through an often complex landscape. Those of us who have been fortunate enough to have an inspirational supervisor will never forget the impact they have had on our practice. They act as an experienced guide leading us through an unfamiliar terrain working with us to reach our destination.

Student nurses place a high value on their practice experience and consider it one of the most important aspects of their pre-registration course. In addition, given that students spend 50 per cent of their time in practice, the relationship they have with their supervisor is central to their development.

Safe preparation of registrants, and others with caring roles, is critical to both patient safety and good patient outcomes. The time you invest in your role as supervisor or assessor, while not always recognised, will have a huge impact on the quality of today's and tomorrow's health professionals. The supervision and assessment of learners is highly valued in today's NHS and the Shape of Caring review highlighted its importance to patient care and safeguarding:

> *This complex role requires support and training. Going beyond teaching knowledge and skills, it involves displaying and modelling leadership attributes. The mentor [as role is referred to in this report] must be conscious of students' individual needs and requirements, and create an atmosphere conducive to learning. Positive role modelling and the opportunity for reflective practice are vital.*

(Willis Commission, 2012, p33)

As a supervisor and/or assessor you will develop both professionally and personally. Professionally, it might be the first step on a teaching pathway and you will be a role model to those around you. It also helps with any future career aspirations as experienced and inspirational supervisors are always valued by employers. You will also develop your confidence and decision-making skills as a result of these activities. Being a supervisor or assessor is a privileged position with the opportunity to impact hugely on student experience and, ultimately, patient care. Given this, we hope you see the importance of the role you are about to embark on for both the current and future workforce.

This chapter will introduce you to the roles and responsibilities for the practice supervisor and practice assessor roles, as well as the NMC *Standards for Student Supervision and Assessment* (NMC, 2018b). We meet Sylvie and Aleksandra in the chapter scenario and consider how the standards apply to their circumstances. You will have an opportunity to consider how reflective practice and models for reflection might enhance your skills as a supervisor/assessor. We then identify and describe 'the team around the student', who may be part of your organisation or other organisations such as a university. The chapter concludes by introducing you to some models used to support learners in practice.

Scenario 1.1

Sylvie is an experienced registrant who works in a community team. She has been working with students as an NMC mentor and has previously undertaken an **NMC-approved** mentor-preparation programme. Working with students is one of her favourite parts of her job and she often finds herself organising learning resources and opportunities for all students within the team. Sylvie is now working with her managers and the link academic from her local university to implement the new NMC *Standards for Student Supervision and Assessment* (NMC, 2018b) within her organisation. She is keen to understand how her mentor experience and qualification will fit with the new practice supervisor and practice assessor roles. Sylvie is working with Aleksandra who has just started her first post with the community team. Aleksandra has had an introduction to how to support learners in practice in the final year of her pre-registration course. She also has lots of experience of being supported as a student herself. Sylvie has been allocated as Aleksandra's preceptor*, and will be supporting her to develop as a practice supervisor.

* A preceptor is an experienced registrant who provides support for new registrants joining the register to help with their transition, for a given period.

This chapter's Scenario 1.1 helps illustrate how influential the roles of supervisor and/or assessor are in today's healthcare environment. We can easily forget the range and longevity of a supervisor or assessor's scope of influence. They are powerful role models and as a result have a huge impact on patient care. Sylvie (Scenario 1.1) has supported many pre-registration students, who themselves have gone on to support a large number of students. Each of those nurses has cared for hundreds of patients; therefore Sylvie's scope of influence is huge. The scenario intends to highlight how valuable the roles of supervisor and assessor are in ensuring high-quality, compassionate care (Pritchard and Gidman, 2012).

In May 2018 the NMC overhauled its standards for supporting and assessing students. This was part of a large-scale review of the NMC *Standards for Education and Training*. The new NMC standards for education and training are split into parts 1 and 2. These are: *Part 1: Standards Framework for Nursing and Midwifery Education* (SFNME) (NMC, 2018d), and *Part 2: Standards for Student Supervision and Assessment* (SSSA) (NMC, 2018b). You may be familiar with the previous standards from pre-2018, and it is likely you will hear terminology from these in your practice setting, especially with regards to the term *mentor*, and this has now been replaced. We begin this chapter by outlining the previous standards to help set the scene and provide some context, before we move into exploring the new standards.

Previous NMC *Standards for Supporting Learning and Assessment in Practice*

In 2018 the NMC *Standards for Supporting Learning and Assessment in Practice* (SLAiP) (NMC, 2008) were replaced. However, the language from them might still be used by colleagues in your organisation. Also, in some areas of this book, we refer to 'mentors' when we outline relevant literature or policy relating to supporting students in the practice area that pre-date the introduction of the new NMC education and training standards in May 2018.

The SLAiP (2008) standards provided a framework that outlined the responsibility of registrants at various points on an educational and student support continuum. These are outlined here as you may find some of your colleagues still referring to these roles, even though they are now outdated.

- The **new registrant** role – while it was expected that every registrant should facilitate learning for students, new registrants, those in the first year of initial registration, were not expected to have any formal role in the assessment of competence of a student, or facilitation of the placement experience.
- **The mentor** – had the remit of providing and facilitating quality learning experiences for students and to assess the student's competence, related to the stage of the course that they are on. To become a mentor you would have undertaken a period of education to support the role, and this course would have been accredited by the NMC. Successful completion of this allowed you to be entered on your organisation's mentor database. Mentors cannot act as a sign-off mentor (see next section).

- **The sign-off mentor** – described experienced mentors who had successfully met additional NMC requirements in order to be able to make judgements about whether a student had achieved the overall standards of competence required for entry onto the register at the end of their NMC-approved programme (NMC, 2010). The employing organisation would have its own process for becoming and achieving sign-off mentor status.
- **Midwifery sign-off mentors** – this mentor would assess the midwifery student at the required level for the clinical placement, in relation to the practice learning outcomes and associated progression points within the NMC-approved programme. As each midwifery clinical placement has a specific set of practice learning outcomes attached to it, all midwifery mentors will be required to have met the additional criteria for sign-off status (this remains the situation until the new midwifery pre-registration standards are released in 2020).
- **Practice teacher** – this described a registrant who was an experienced NMC mentor, and who had then undertaken additional education incorporating the NMC (2008) practice teacher competencies. All students undertaking a programme leading to registration as a specialist community public health nurse (SCPHN) needed a named practice teacher. The practice teacher status was recorded on a local register and they were required to undertake a triennial review.
- **The NMC teacher** – this described a registrant who undertook an NMC-approved teacher preparation programme to achieve the knowledge, skills and competence required to support learning and assessment for students on NMC-approved programmes. They were usually based in a higher education institution, and this qualification was recorded on the NMC register.

The SLAiP standards used the term mentor to define a registrant who *facilitates learning and supervises and assesses students in a practice setting* (NMC, 2008, p45). All nursing and midwifery students on pre-registration programmes were provided with a designated mentor for the duration of their placement. The mentor would work closely with their student and have responsibility for both the supervision of practice as well as the assessment of the student. The SSSA replaces the mentor role with two distinct roles of the practice supervisor and practice assessor. In addition, the NMC recognises that the practice supervisor can be any registered health and social care professional who facilitates and supports students with their practice learning where appropriate. The SLAiP (2008) standards required mentors to undertake an NMC-approved preparation course before individuals could take on this role. This often led to waiting lists for potential mentors wanting to access such a course, and could then impact the potential mentor numbers of a placement area. The SSSA recognises that preparation for the supervisor and assessor role is best governed by the employing organisation, working in collaboration with the student's approved educational institution (AEI). Concerns have been raised about the quality of mentorship and assessment being variable in the old model. Also, there is a potential for a lack of objectivity in the assessment of students whom mentors have become very familiar with, leading to students passing when perhaps they should have failed. This increases the risk of *failing to fail,* a term derived from Kathleen Duffy's (2003) work, and discussed further in Chapter 7.

The *Standards Framework for Nursing and Midwifery Education*

The new *Standards Framework for Nursing and Midwifery Education* (NMC, 2018d) has now replaced the SLAiP (NMC, 2008) and comprises three parts:

- *Part 1: Standards Framework for Nursing and Midwifery Education;*
- *Part 2: Standards for Student Supervision and Assessment;*
- *Part 3: Programme Standards – for pre-registration nursing education and prescribing programmes.*

It is Part 2, the *Standards for Student Supervision and Assessment* (SSSA), that we will look at in more detail throughout this book as these set out the *expectations for the learning, support and supervision of students in the practice environment.* They also outline how students are assessed for both theory and practice (NMC, 2018b, p3).

The SSSA are for all *NMC-approved* education programmes and as such they relate to all fields of nursing, midwifery, specialist community public health nursing and those undertaking NMC-approved prescribing programmes, for example. They will also cover Nursing Associate (NA) programmes, as the role becomes regulated by the NMC from early 2019. The SSSA retains the supernumerary status of students and states they *must be supported to learn without being counted as part of the staffing required for safe and effective care* (NMC, 2018b, p4). There is also reference to the supernumerary status of apprentices studying an NMC-approved programme with an integrated apprenticeship route. In relation to these students the standards state that: *this includes practice placements within their place of employment; this does not apply when they are working in their substantive role* (p4). The SSSA comprises three broad headings and ten sections. This book covers each of these areas in detail, but this next section presents an overview of the main areas to familiarise you with the underpinning principles and requirements.

Effective practice learning – focuses on providing safe and effective learning opportunities for student nurses and midwives when engaged in practice-based learning. There is a requirement for AEIs and practice-learning partners to work together to ensure that all the standards for supervision and assessment of students are met. One way of facilitating this is by nominating an individual to be responsible for actively supporting students and addressing any concerns. This is a requirement of the SSSA and this role may have a range of titles such as **Learning environment manager** – in addition, students must be given the opportunity to learn from a range of people, including service users and other students. This emphasis on learning beyond the supervisor is welcomed and should also open up opportunities to learn from a range of professionals.

Another requirement, which again moves away from over-reliance on the student–supervisor relationship, is that all NMC registrants must actively contribute to practice learning. Therefore, it is everyone's business, not just those with a defined role or those who have been allocated as a supervisor or assessor. Learning opportunities and experiences should not be a *one size fits all* approach. They should be tailored to meet the students' needs, for example taking into account the programme they are on, where they are in the programme and the proficiencies they need to meet during the placement. Students should be encouraged to work with practice colleagues to construct and evaluate these opportunities and experiences; not just for themselves but for others. Evaluation and feedback of learning is an underpinning principle of good educational practice and something all supervisors and assessors should be engaged in.

Supervision of students – the new SSSA separates the roles of supervisor and assessor. Previously, these roles were combined into the mentor role. This separation is intended to increase objectivity and therefore lead to more robust assessment processes and decisions. According to the SSSA, practice supervisors may be an NMC registrant but may also be another type of registered health and social care professional (e.g. Health and Care Professions Council, General Pharmaceutical Council or General Medical Council). If they are an NMC registrant they do not need to be on the same part of the register, or same field of nursing as the student they are supervising. However, they must support learning in line with their *scope of practice* (this is explained in Table 1.1).

You may have heard colleagues being confused as to the role of the supervisor in assessing students. Supervisors may also be assessors (if they meet the criteria) – but cannot be supervising and assessing the same student. The roles are clearly separated. However, a supervisor must contribute to the assessment of the students' achievement of proficiency. What this means is that their written and verbal feedback, which is based on a number of observations, discussion and simulation, etc., must be taken into account by the assessor when making judgements about achievement of proficiencies and progression or completion. If the supervisor has concerns about a student's competence or **fitness to practise**, they should raise this with the practice assessor and the academic linking to the practice area from the student's AEI. There must be adequate opportunity to discuss these concerns.

Another potential area of major change for practice colleagues regarding the practice supervisor role is around the preparation for the role. Previously, all registrants supporting students on NMC-approved programmes needed to have completed an NMC-approved mentor preparation programme. This is no longer the case for supervisors. The SSSA states supervisors must be given ongoing support to prepare, reflect and develop effective supervision and contribution to student learning and assessment. In addition, they need to be knowledgeable of the programme the student they are supervising is undertaking and any proficiencies they are required to meet. This means that your organisation will have its own preparation for the practice supervisor role arrangements in place, usually designed with the AEI that your organisation takes students from. Activity 1.1 will help to explore this further.

Activity 1.1   Critical thinking

In Scenario 1.1 we met Aleksandra, a newly qualified registrant who requires preparation to become a practice supervisor in her clinical area. Aleksandra is a child field nurse working in a child and adolescent mental health community team. This is a popular and busy student placement area, which accepts students from all fields of nursing, midwifery students and also other students, including physiotherapy and occupational therapy. Aleksandra is interested to know which students she can supervise.

Given what you have learnt already about the SSSA:

- Can Aleksandra be a practice supervisor?
- If so, which students can she supervise?
- Would she be able to make assessment decisions about a student's achievement of proficiencies?

There is a model answer for this activity at the end of this chapter.

You will have noted from Activity 1.1 that the character Aleksandra from Scenario 1.1 would require preparation and support for the role of practice supervisor. The NMC (2018b) states the preparation for this role should include opportunities for supervisors to:

- receive ongoing support to prepare, reflect and develop for effective supervision and contribution to student learning and assessment; and
- have understanding of the proficiencies and programme outcomes they are supporting students to achieve.

Practice assessors require different support and preparation for this role. Chapter 5 of this book explores preparation requirements for these roles in more detail.

Assessment of students and confirmation of proficiency – this section of the new standards focuses on the responsibilities of those colleagues who are assessing either academic or practice achievement. These roles are now more clearly defined and there is a requirement that the assessors have a greater distance from the students' day-to-day support, to increase the rigour of assessment decisions. The SSSA includes the requirement for students to be assigned a new academic assessor for each part of the programme. This role is for academic staff in the student's AEI. This means that with regards to a pre-registration undergraduate registrant degree programme, students would need a different academic assessor for Years 1, 2 and 3. These new requirements in the SSSA have the intention to make all assessment decisions more robust and objective. You may be familiar with previous practice in your clinical setting where students have a different practice mentor/assessor for each placement.

The criteria about which students a registrant can act as assessor for are more pre-scriptive than those applied to the supervisor role. Examples of how the criteria might manifest in practice are modelled in Table 1.1

Type of student	Type of assessor	Can they assess?
Nursing student adult field	Registered nurse adult field	Yes
Nursing student – mental health field	Registered nurse – child field, working in child and adolescent setting	Yes Assessor is a registered nurse with appropriate equivalent experience for the student's field of practice
Nursing student – child field	Registered nurse – mental health field, working in an older adult dementia assessment unit	No Although the registrant is a registered nurse and suitably prepared to carry out the assessor role they are not child field nor do they have appropriate equivalent experience working with children
Midwifery student	Registered midwife	Yes The practice and academic assessors must be registered midwives
Specialist community public health nurse (health visiting) student	Specialist community public health nurse (school nursing) student working in a 0–19 service	Yes Registered SCPHN and appropriate equivalent experience of children and young people
Nursing student – learning disability field	Academic assessor is a registered nurse mental health field	No The academic does not have appropriate equivalent experience in learning disabilities

Table 1.1 Applying the NMC assessor criteria

In addition to the criteria presented in Table 1.1, practice assessors must maintain *current knowledge and expertise* (NMC, 2018b, p9) for the proficiencies and programme outcomes they are assessing. The practice assessor must work with the academic assessor when recommending the student for progression to the next part of the programme. Let's apply some of the criteria to the characters from Scenario 1.1. Sylvie is an NMC registrant (mental health field), she has previously completed an NMC-approved mentor-preparation course, therefore she is eligible to assess pre-registration students. However, she must have the appropriate equivalent experience for the student's field of practice. That may have been gained as a result of her own field of practice being the same as that of the student she is assessing. Additionally, this may be because of the experience she has gained through her professional experience.

Practice assessors must base their assessment decisions in part on direct observation of the students and must not rely solely on feedback from others. However, they do need to collect feedback from others, including supervisors as well as testimonies from patients and service users. By doing this, they are able to triangulate information from different sources to help them make more reliable decisions. Also, the NMC is clear that a practice assessor cannot also be that student's practice supervisor, although they may be simultaneously supervising other students who they are not assessing. This all adds to objectivity in the assessment process. Assessment issues are covered in more detail in Chapter 6.

Practice assessors also require preparation for the role. They may be new to assessing students or they may have previously successfully completed an NMC-approved mentor preparation programme. However experienced they are in supporting learners in practice, they need to demonstrate the following:

- interpersonal communication skills;
- conducting objective and evidence based assessment of students;
- providing constructive feedback to facilitate professional development of others;
- knowledge of the assessment process and their role in it.

So how can an NMC registrant achieve this? If you have previously completed an NMC-approved mentor course like Sylvie in Scenario 1.1, then that will meet the criteria above. However, if you have not then you must be able to evidence the above. This may be through continuing professional development activities related to the above outcomes. This can be evidenced with an established practice assessor or your line manager during your appraisal. Alternatively, you may complete an *assessor preparation course* delivered by your organisation or local AEI. This course will not be approved by the NMC as there is no requirement for this under the new SSSA. It will, however, provide you with an opportunity to explore assessment and related issues, in more detail. In addition to any preparation for the role, practice assessors and supervisors must: have access to ongoing support and training for the role; demonstrate continued professional development (which is a requirement of revalidation) and be familiar with programme proficiencies and outcomes of the programme on which the student they are assessing is enrolled.

Activity 1.2 Critical thinking

In Scenario 1.1 we met Sylvie who is an experienced registrant who works in a community team. She has been working with students as an NMC mentor and has previously undertaken an NMC-approved mentor-preparation programme.

Given what you have learnt already about the SSSA (NMC, 2018b) and the SLAiP standards (NMC, 2008):

1. Can Sylvie be a practice supervisor?
2. Can Sylvie be a practice assessor?
3. What information from the scenario informed your answers?

There is a model answer for this activity at the end of this chapter.

You might find your colleagues and organisation still refer to the roles from the SLAiP standards (NMC, 2008). In particular the *mentor* term is frequently used when discussing supporting learners in practice, and has been associated with supporting students for decades. You might have an opportunity to become involved in implementing the SSSA in your particular clinical area. This is an exciting time, being able to shape how the new roles are embedded into practice. The role of adequately prepared supervisors and assessors of clinical practice remains critical in facilitating the development of future generations of nurses and midwives.

Using reflective practice in your role

Reflecting on your practice is an essential aspect of nursing and midwifery. There is widespread recognition of the value of reflection and reflective practice. It helps to develop practice and enhances our ability to learn from and through experiences. It also supports us to manage the psychological demands of care delivery. Reflection is essential in helping us consider quality aspects of care and areas for improvement. It helps those supporting practice learning to be aware of their own knowledge, skills and beliefs about students; learning; teaching and assessment. Analysing and thinking about our supervision and assessment experiences provides a natural opportunity to deepen our skills. Howatson-Jones (2016) offers a really useful guide if you are interested in reading further about what reflection is, why it is so important and how to use it in your practice.

Reflective models can help guide us with our reflective practice. A simple reflective cycle is suggested by Gibbs (1988). It is iterative and cyclical in that Gibbs suggests we learn by repeating our experiences. The model has the following six stages:

1. Description
2. Feelings

3. Evaluation

4. Analysis

5. Conclusion

6. Action plans

Gibbs' model is commonly used within the health professions as it is clear and precise. It allows for description, analysis and evaluation of an experience to help an individual make sense of experiences and practice. Reflecting on its own is not enough; you then have to put into practice the learning and new understanding you have gained. This ensures the learning from the reflective process informs your future practice (Gibbs, 1988). There are many models available to guide reflection, and Gibbs' model is just one of those. As with any model, choose one that you find fits your particular style. Using models can help us master reflective practice and ensure we complete the whole cycle. Taking action is essential and reflective models prompt the individual to formulate an action plan. This enables the reflective practitioner to look at their practice and see what they would change in the future, how they would develop/improve their practice. The further reading at the end of this chapter directs you to other reflective models if you are interested in finding out more. The centrality of reflection to the profession is further mirrored in revalidation requirements (NMC, 2017a). It is therefore unsurprising that being reflective as a practice supervisor and/or assessor is essential. Activity 1.3 offers an opportunity to critically think about reflecting on practice as we are presented with a draft of a reflection form completed by Sylvie, from Scenario 1.1.

Activity 1.3   Critical thinking

In Scenario 1.1 we met Sylvie. She has been reflecting on a practice experience as part of her evidence for her upcoming **NMC revalidation**, using Gibbs' model (1988). The experience she has chosen is her involvement in developing a workbook for new practice supervisors in her organisation.

Please read through this draft of her reflection form. 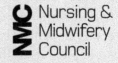 Nursing & Midwifery Council

REFLECTIVE ACCOUNTS FORM

You must use this form to record five written reflective accounts on your CPD and/or practice-related feedback and/or an event or experience in your practice and how this relates to the Code. Please fill in a page for each of your reflective accounts, making sure you do not include any information that might identify a specific patient, service user or colleague. Please refer to our guidance on preserving anonymity in the section on non-identifiable information in **How to revalidate with the NMC**.

Reflective account:

What was the nature of the CPD activity and/or practice-related feedback and/or event or experience in your practice?

1. **Description**

I have been involved in developing a workbook to prepare colleagues to become practice supervisors for students. I have worked with others involved in supporting learners in practice, including community colleagues, managers and academics from the University. We also had students working with us to help us focus the content. We have had several meetings over the past six months and each taken responsibility to develop part of the workbook. The final workbook is now completed and has been signed off for use by the Trust management team. We are starting to use it and I have offered to evaluate the workbook over the next six months.

2. **Feelings**

I felt apprehensive at first when I read the new *Standards for Student Supervision and Assessment* (NMC, 2018) as I could not imagine how we could 'lose' the mentor role. Mentoring is a big part of my professional identity and at first, I felt like I didn't want to give up this title. However, I was really pleased to be asked to take part in this work as I feel I have lots of experience from my previous mentor role, which I was able to share and use for this workbook. I was also pleased to be part of a bigger team working on this and I enjoyed working with colleagues from different backgrounds.

What did you learn from the CPD activity and/or feedback and/or event or experience in your practice?

3. **Evaluation**

The new NMC *Standards for Student Supervision and Assessment* (2018) have overhauled the previous standards and part of this has meant scrapping the mentor role. Instead, we are having two other roles to support learners. Organisations are free to decide who is best suited

---

(Continued)

(Continued)

to supervising and assessing students, as well as how they are prepared for these roles. The new standards should ensure students can be supervised at all times and by a range of registrants, rather than waiting for their designated mentor to become free.

This provides an opportunity for new staff to be practice supervisors and we need to be able to prepare them for this important role. We have developed a workbook that is easily accessible and can prepare any nursing, midwifery or allied health professional registrant who is interested in supporting students as a *practice supervisor*. Creating a workbook means we can support more staff in a timelier manner, rather than waiting for a place on a mentor course. It's important to be working **multi-professionally** on these sorts of initiatives, as that's how we are expecting our students to be able to work.

4. **Analysis**

We have had lots of colleagues inputting into this and worked in a collaborative way (Tasselli, 2015). I think this has really added to the quality of the workbook and hopefully has helped get others on board. Involving students as well has really helped to gain a focus on what's important for this role (Haraldseid et al., 2016). This has shaped my commitment to involve other colleagues, professions and students in the evaluation. I now feel less anxious about the changes and I have had time to really get to know the new standards (NMC, 2018) and think about what this means to practice.

How did you change or improve your practice as a result?

5. **Conclusion**

I have learnt that by creating a workbook we can support more staff in a timelier manner, rather than waiting for a place on a mentor course. It's important to be working multi-professionally on these sorts of initiatives, as that's how we are expecting our students to be able to work. I have also learnt that being involved in shaping and designing part of my organisation's implementation of the *Standards for Student Supervision and Assessment* (NMC, 2018) has helped me better understand the standards and allay any anxieties I had. Although I might feel anxious about a change involving my 'mentor status' getting involved in the workbook has helped me to feel more in control about the changes and be more prepared for my new practice supervisor and practice assessor roles.

---

6.   **Action plans**

How is this relevant to the Code?

Select one or more themes: Prioritise people – Practise effectively – Preserve safety – Promote professionalism and trust

---

Once you have read Sylvie's draft reflection:

1.   Complete an action plan for Sylvie.
2.   Look at the last section of the form and consider how this is relevant to the Code (NMC, 2015). You can read the Code online at **www.nmc.org. uk/standards/code/read-the-code-online**.

There is a model answer at the end of this chapter.

You may wish to share your reflections with your peers or manager during appraisal. Maybe you noted in Activity 1.3 that often actions from reflections involve sharing information with others. You could reflect upon supporting a learner's experience with others who you know have been involved in supporting a particular student. This offers an opportunity to learn with and from others. As Sylvie (from Scenario 1.1) will have found from her engagement with the SSSA and her involvement in developing the workbook, there is a wider team involved in supporting learners in practice.

The wider team involved in supporting the student

In today's world of interprofessional education and working, and outcomes-focused patient care, a team approach to supporting student learning is essential. We have already learnt from the SSSA (NMC, 2018b) that other registered health professionals can act as practice supervisors for our students. We also know that the practice assessor is a separate role to supervisor, so already there are a minimum of two individuals supporting a student's learning in the clinical area. However, if we start to consider others from within our organisation whose role it is to support placement learning, along with those supporting from the student's AEI, we start to see the scale of potential support available. Figure 1.1 illustrates examples of potential support available to students while on placement. Studies have found that the best support teams are diverse teams – diverse in disciplines, professions, knowledge and abilities, as well as age, gender, background, life experiences, among others. Diversity represents different viewpoints and can help students make better decisions, find better solutions and produce better outcomes than individual experts working alone or groups of homogeneous experts (Whitelock et al., 2015).

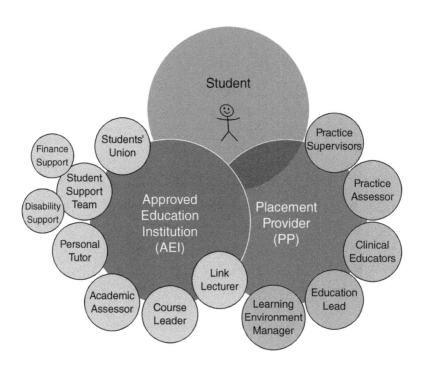

Figure 1.1 Examples of potential support available to students while on placement

Figure 1.1 represents the triad arrangement of support involving the student, placement providers (PPs) and AEIs. They all work collaboratively to support learning throughout the student's pre-registration programme. You may already be aware of colleagues in your practice area whose role it is to support placement learning. Although these vary within organisations, they could include other practice supervisors and/or assessors, managers and education leads. There also exists a support network for the student from the student's AEI. These might include the student's personal tutor, designated student support staff and course leaders. Table 1.2 outlines common roles you might come across, involved with supporting the student in the clinical area, as well as the types of support that they could offer. Please note these roles will vary depending on the organisational requirements.

The link lecturer role has long been associated with support for student nurses and midwives in clinical practice. It is worth further consideration as it is critically placed to bridge the gap between clinical practice and AEIs in supporting students. The NMC

Roles	Definition and support offered
Practice supervisors	*Any registrant within the practice area who has been suitably prepared and supported to undertake the practice supervisor role.*
	Can support students by being a practice supervisor.
	Can help you to develop your skills; support you with your development; provide a different viewpoint and/or advice on student learning matters.
Practice assessors	*Any NMC registrant within the practice area who is an experienced supervisor and has been suitably prepared and supported to undertake the practice assessor role.*
	Can support students by being a practice assessor.
	Can help you to develop your skills; support you with your development; provide a different viewpoint and/or advice on student learning matters.
Learning environment managers (LEMs)	*Usually a registrant based in each placement area who has a particular interest in supporting students in practice, and takes on additional related duties.*
	Can support students by directing them to learning resources and opportunities in the practice area.
	May allocate students to practice supervisors and/or practice assessors for the practice area. Will undertake the practice area educational audit and co-ordinates student evaluations for the area.
	Can help you to develop your skills; support you with your development; provide a different viewpoint and/or advice on student learning matters.
Clinical educators/ practice educators/ professional development leads	*Often expert practitioners from a clinical area, likely to have responsibility for training and development duties across a department or clinical speciality.*
	Can support students by directing them to learning opportunities and wider networks of learners.
	Can help you to develop your skills; support you with your development; provide a different viewpoint and/or advice on student learning matters.
Education lead/director of education	*A senior figure within an organisation or department. The role likely to involve: managing education provision across an organisation or area planning, delivering and evaluating a range of programmes to meet strategic and operational needs; working with a range of staff to identify future education requirements and providing advice on provision; providing advice to the organisation on improving the quality of education.*
	Supports students by strategically working to plan placement experiences across the organisation. Working in partnership with AEIs and supporting curriculum development.
	Can support you by providing training and development opportunities to further your skills and by providing networking opportunities for you to meet with other supervisors/assessors and lecturers.

(Continued)

Table 1.2 (Continued)

Roles	Definition and support offered
Link lecturer/ placement support	*Employed and based at an AEI as an academic. The role commonly involves a point of connection between the AEI and placement area to support student's practice-based learning.*
	Supports the student by being the contact for the AEI while on placement, assisting with issues and queries.
	Can support you with student issues and queries; assessment and failing matters; quality processes; your professional development.
Course leader/ programme leader/course director	*Employed and based at an AEI as an academic with the responsibility for academic leadership, management and assessment, for the course they have been designated to lead on.*
	Supports the student by responding to feedback from students, external examiners, Professional, Statutory and Regulatory Bodies (PSRBs) and industry.
	Can support you by providing updates and workshops and involving you in educational and curriculum development opportunities, to help your professional development.
Personal tutor/ academic advisor	*Employed and based at an AEI as an academic with the remit of providing academic and professional development support to their allocated students.*
	Supports students to make decisions in relation to their course, formulate plans to support their academic and personal/professional development. They connect the student with other academics and opportunities as well as with other support services as appropriate.
	Can support you with particular student issues by providing further information about the student as appropriate, or signposting the student to other services and processes.
Academic assessor	*Employed and based at an AEI as an academic with the NMC remit of reviewing the student's performance with regards to their achievement of proficiencies and programme learning outcomes prior to progression.*
	Will not have a role in supervising the student in practice, teaching, assessing theoretical work or as an academic advisor for the student for the part of the programme being assessed. However, they will meet with the student at course progression points.
	Can communicate with practice assessors about assessment decisions relating to progression.
Student support services/ student support officers/ pastoral support	*Employed and based at an AEI to provide confidential, impartial help and support to students, prospective students and graduates.*
	Supports the student by signposting to specialised support services including: student help; student funding; international student; careers and employability; disabled student access; wellbeing and multi-faith. Can also support the student with AEI processes, for example absence monitoring and assessment submission.
	Can support you by directing your student to specialised services.

Roles	Definition and support offered
Students' Union	*Organisation that promotes, defends and extends the rights of students.* Supports the student by offering a professional, impartial, confidential and non-judgemental service, providing advice, support and representation to help resolve problems. Also provides networking opportunities, access to societies and clubs, friendship groups, extra curricula opportunities that can develop employability skills. Can support you by directing your student to specialised services.

Table 1.2   Roles involved in supporting the student in the clinical area

SLAiP standards (NMC, 2008) suggested the link role should account for a maximum of 20 per cent of the university-based registrant's remit to allow them to keep up to date. However, registrant lecturers have always been supported by the NMC to use other means to keep them updated if they didn't undertake a link role. There has been a long-standing academic discussion about the value of the link lecturer role as there is little consistency regarding its purpose, objective and contribution to practice-based learning (MacIntosh, 2015).

The new SSSA (NMC, 2018b) has removed the requirement of registrant teacher qualification and thus the future of the link lecturer role is increasingly unclear. If AEIs choose to keep this role and use registrant lecturers in a more strategic remit, the role has the potential to flourish. In particular, the value of this role could be in helping consistent and timely communications by being the 'face' of the AEI for busy practitioners in practice. Some AEIs might use the link lecturer role to fulfil the NMC academic assessor role requirements. They can also support the preparation and continued professional development of supervisors and assessors, and provide a valuable link to the students' curricula.

The range and breadth of individuals involved in student support also provides a depth in the types of support that can be offered. Different individuals specialise in particular aspects of support, e.g. financial support, and they are there to advise the student and us as supervisors accordingly. This should remind us as practice supervisors and/ or assessors that we are just one part of a larger team. We shouldn't ever feel out of our depth as we have numerous other individuals around us to help with any student requests, issues or situations that we are unable to handle.

Students benefit from this wider network of support as they can learn from multiple perspectives and combine ideas to develop with their studies. Practice supervisors and/ or assessors also benefit from opportunities to connect and learn from others. Sylvie, the character introduced in Scenario 1.1, makes use of a wider network to help her to develop different perspectives on the workbook content (Activity 1.3). Supporting students as a team embeds and establishes a collaborative culture that is required for achieving the goal of student progression.

Models of organising student support in practice areas

There is a shortage of qualified nurses and midwives in the UK, as well as in many other countries. The shortage is likely to be made more challenging in future years due to the cap on spending on agency staff, the reduction in overseas recruitment and changes to student funding. This has an effect on the ambitious plans to deliver healthcare as policies set out. As well as the NMC revising the way student nurses and midwives should be supported in clinical practice in the SSSA (NMC, 2018b), there have also been other drivers to develop new models of student support. An example is in the NHS *Five Year Forward View*, which was published in October 2014 by NHS England, and sets out a new shared vision for the future of the NHS based around the new models of care. However, in order to develop a workforce that is responsive to changes in care, now and in the future, there is a need to ensure there is a sufficient supply of highly skilled staff.

> *We can design innovative new care models, but they simply won't become a reality unless we have a workforce with the right numbers, skills, values and behaviours to deliver it.*

(NHS England, 2014, p29)

It is therefore important to reduce attrition, or student drop out, from pre-registration programmes. Of equal importance is ensuring that the students who graduate are resilient and are recruited and retained in the workforce. Organisations and education providers have begun to work together differently to attract and retain the right students and to ensure they provide a high-quality clinical learning environment. This requirement is also reflected in *Raising the Bar: Shape of Caring: A Review of the Future Education and Training of Registered Nurses and Care Assistants* (Willis, 2015).

A large-scale project across Health Education England (HEE) in the East of the region set out to improve the quality and capacity of the practice learning environments. Relevant publications relating to placement support and clinical learning were reviewed and from this a number of new approaches were developed and piloted in different organisations. One of these that has been evaluated and findings disseminated, is the Collaborative Learning in Practice (CLiP) model. Perhaps you work in an area where this has been piloted?

CLiP is based on a concept of coaching where the focus is on developing students' confidence, competence and performance through practice support. Students are expected to take responsibility for their learning and their coach encourages them to identify their own learning needs and requirements. The coach has the responsibility for the quality of the learning experience (Lobo et al., 2014). This model supports the SSSA (NMC, 2018b) as the 'coach' and 'practice supervisor' are a similar role.

A practice assessor steps in at the relevant assessment points, but the supervisor is responsible for the day-to-day learning.

From the evaluations of the models available to date (Clarke et al., 2018), it seems that there are six common principles in these new and emerging approaches to organising student support in practice areas:

1. A coaching approach is useful.
2. Support should be provided by a team – responsibility for practice learning and assessment decisions should not be only with one individual.
3. Students should be delivering hands-on care – supervisors supporting the student to provide care is at the heart of new approaches.
4. Strong leadership is required for sustained change.
5. New approaches require a sustainable infrastructure.
6. Linking pre-registration education and workforce supply directly into an organisation's business agenda is helpful to maintain the profile.

CLiP has been adopted in many areas, and it is important to note that other models of organising placement learning also exist. Perhaps you have been involved in your practice setting with trying out new ways of organising student support? Activity 1.4 provides an opportunity for you to identify student support mechanisms in your own clinical practice area.

Activity 1.4   Leadership and management reflection

Each organisation will have its own unique approach to organising student support. As a practice supervisor and/or assessor, it is critical you recognise mechanisms for organising student support in your area.

1. Look at *Figure 1.1 Examples of potential support available to students while on placement.* Consider the student support network for your own practice area. It will be helpful for you to make a note of this for your future reference.
2. Consider which (if any) models of organising student support exist or might be useful in your practice area.*

* You may need to speak to experienced colleagues in your practice area to help you with this activity.

There is no model answer for this activity as it relates to your own experience.

It is clear that there is a need to explore different ways of supporting students to ensure they have high-quality learning experiences without compromising patient safety and patient care. In Activity 1.4 you will have identified approaches to organising student support in your own practice setting. CLiP and many other models of supporting students seem to have a common element of having a coaching approach. Coaching fits well with the new SSSA (NMC, 2018b). Coaching is well established in the sporting world, and describes a relationship where someone trains others through instructing them and giving them advice. In relation to practice-based education, the term describes an interactive and facilitative process where a student is supported to acquire and develop skills and abilities needed for their profession by an experienced registrant over a given time period (Kelton, 2014). If you are interested in exploring coaching methods and how these could enhance your practice supervisor and/or assessor role, check out the book by Cox et al. (2014). Details are provided in the further reading section of this chapter.

Chapter summary

This chapter has introduced you to the role and responsibilities for the practice supervisor and practice assessor roles. These are new roles emerging from the recently published NMC SSSA (NMC, 2018b) which has replaced the SLAiP (NMC, 2008). These new standards bring with them many changes, which have been introduced in this chapter, and will feature throughout this book. Through meeting Sylvie and Aleksandra in the chapter scenario, and the chapter activities, we have attempted to bring these new NMC standards to life by applying them to a range of situations. The chapter included some consideration of how reflective practice and reflective models might enhance your skills as a supervisor and/or assessor. In particular, we looked at how Sylvie had used Gibbs' model (1988) to guide her reflective practice and to help her structure her reflective account to be used towards her NMC revalidation (2017a). The wider team supporting student practice learning was identified with reference to common roles that you are likely to encounter. The chapter concluded with consideration of some new and emerging models of organising student support in practice areas.

Activity answers

Activity 1.1: Critical thinking (p8)

1.   It is not clear whether Aleksandra has been suitably prepared to take on the role of practice supervisor. She would need preparation for the role, as guided by her employing organisation. It is likely that Sylvie will support her preparation for the role, as Sylvie is an experienced mentor and preceptor. She would need to work with Sylvie and other colleagues to identify opportunities to reflect on her role as supervisor and to enable her to develop in this role. Furthermore, she would need to have an

understanding of the proficiencies and programme outcomes for the students she supervises.

2. If she meets the criteria outlined above, she can supervise the full range of pre-registration students.

3. Aleksandra cannot make decisions about a student's achievement of proficiencies as this is the role of the practice assessor. However, her feedback of the student's competence should be taken into account by the assessor and used to make judgements about achievement and progression.

Activity 1.2: Critical thinking (pp10–11)

1 & 2. Yes, it is likely from the scenario that Sylvie could be a practice supervisor and a practice assessor. However, in accordance with the SSSA, she would not be able to act as a supervisor to those students she is allocated to assess.

3. As we know that Sylvie has previously completed an NMC-approved mentor course, and is already an experienced mentor, this will have prepared her to act in either of the roles. However, she will need to have access to ongoing support and training for the roles; demonstrate she undertakes continued professional development and be familiar with programme proficiencies and outcomes of the students she is assessing.

Activity 1.3: Critical thinking (pp12–15)

1. Question 1: You may have noted some or all of these activities for Sylvie's action plan.

- Evaluate the workbook – The final workbook is completed and has been signed off for use by the Trust's management team. Sylvie has offered to evaluate the workbook over the next six months.
- Staff development – As part of the developing team, we can assume Sylvie would be involved in working with colleagues on how to use the workbook.
- Disseminate the findings – As part of the developing team, we can assume Sylvie would talk to colleagues in her organisation about the new workbook and how it has been developed. As part of her role in the evaluation, she would be required to disseminate the findings of the evaluation through a report, and potentially through presentations or publications.
- Networking – Sylvie will need to carry on working with others as part of the evaluation and to be able to continually develop the workbook.

2. Question 2: You may have noted some or all of these standards from Sylvie's reflection.

- 6 – Always practise in line with the best available evidence.
- 7 – Communicate clearly.
- 8 – Work cooperatively.
- 9 – Share your skills, knowledge and experience for the benefit of people receiving care and your colleagues.
- 20 – Uphold the reputation of your profession at all times.
- 22 – Fulfil all registration requirements.

Further reading

Howatson-Jones, L (2016) *Reflective Practice in Nursing*. London: Sage/Learning Matters.

This book supports the reader in discovering how you can apply principles of reflection to enhance your practice, patient care and professional development.

Cox, E, Bachkirova, T and Clutterbuck, DA (eds) (2014) *The Complete Handbook of Coaching.* London: Sage.

This book provides a useful guide to coaching that can be applied to a range of different professions and settings. It is aimed at helping new coaches develop their own personal style of coaching, building on approaches explained from coaching theory.

Useful websites

Supporting information on *Standards for Student Supervision and Assessment* (SISSSA) NMC 2018 **www.nmc.org.uk/supporting-information-on-standards-for-student-supervision-and-assessment/**

These pages contain the supporting information for all the NMC new information supporting the new standards relating to student supervision and assessment. Please familiarise yourself with these and in particular the guides to the roles which the NMC are developing as a quick and accessible reference point. It is updated regularly.

Chapter 2   Learning culture

(Continued)

9.3 deal with differences of professional opinion with colleagues by discussion and informed debate, respecting their views and opinions and behaving in a professional way at all times, and

9.4 support students' and colleagues' learning to help them develop their professional competence and confidence.

11.1 only delegate tasks and duties that are within the other person's scope of competence, making sure that they fully understand your instructions.

11.2 make sure that everyone you delegate tasks to is adequately supervised and supported so they can provide safe and compassionate care.

11.3 confirm that the outcome of any task you have delegated to someone else meets the required standard.

Preserve safety

15.3 take account of your own safety, the safety of others and the availability of other options for providing care.

16. act without delay if you believe that there is a risk to patient safety or public protection (16.1–16.6).

19.1 take measures to reduce as far as possible, the likelihood of mistakes, near misses, harm and the effect of harm if it takes place.

19.2 take account of current evidence, knowledge and developments in reducing mistakes and the effect of them and the impact of human factors and system failures (see the note below).

19.4 take all reasonable personal precautions necessary to avoid any potential health risks to colleagues, people receiving care and the public.

Promote professionalism and trust

20. uphold the reputation of your profession at all times (20.1–20.10).

21.1 refuse all but the most trivial gifts, favours or hospitality as accepting them could be interpreted as an attempt to gain preferential treatment.

22 fulfil all registration requirements (22.1–22.3).

23.1 cooperate with any audits of training records, registration records or other relevant audits that we may want to carry out to make sure you are still fit to practise.

23.3 tell any employers you work for if you have had your practice restricted or had any other conditions imposed on you by us or any other relevant body.

25.2 support any staff you may be responsible for to follow the Code at all times. They must have the knowledge, skills and competence for safe practice; and understand how to raise any concerns linked to any circumstances where the Code has, or could be, broken.

Chapter aims

After reading this chapter, you will be able to:

- understand how to create and maintain a safe learning environment for patients and students;
- describe what makes a good learning environment and placement learning experience;
- identify the role yourself and others play in valuing the learning environment and creating opportunities for collaboration;
- accommodate a diverse range of students into your practice area.

This chapter begins by looking at the increasingly diverse range of students in practice areas. We meet Jethro, an experienced supervisor in a community team, who is supporting a number of different students. We move on to consider students' individual needs, including those with a disability who may need additional support while on placement. Then we focus on the standards that relate to governance: these are *creating and maintaining a safe learning environment* and *valuing the learning environment*. The chapter concludes by considering how you can effectively use the evidence to enhance your effectiveness as a supervisor or assessor.

The diversification of students

Registered nurses have a history of supporting a wide range of students in practice including student nurses, student midwives and ex-registrants who are wishing to *return to practice* (Health Education England, no date). However, greater diversification of the healthcare workforce is underway, and more is planned, both within and outside the nursing profession. You may already be working with new types of healthcare workers and over the next years you will see the arrival of a wider range of colleagues such as nurse associates, assistant practitioners, nurse apprentices, advanced clinical practitioners and physician associates (Miller et al., 2015). To add to this, nursing students now fund their course fees and are no longer eligible for a bursary to support them with living expenses. They now access student loans like any other student (HM Treasury, 2015). This change in funding from commissioned to self-funder may have an impact on how they perceive their role as a student nurse and their expectations of both their placement experience and the support they receive from their supervisors and assessors. Therefore, you will need to be adaptable and demonstrate resilience in order to successfully support this range of students. Activity 2.1 offers you the opportunity to think about the students in your practice area.

Activity 2.1   Critical thinking

Who's who in your clinical area?

Take a look around your clinical area; you may be working on a ward, out-patient clinic, a community setting or in primary care. Notice how many and what types of students access your clinical area. Make a list and identify if they are already registrants (e.g. advanced clinical practitioners); their disciplines; where they are in their student journey and whether they are preparing to become one of the new types of healthcare workers such as physician associates. Are they studying for a traditional degree or an apprenticeship? Finally, where are they studying and what courses?

Now think about your colleagues and consider their role and responsibilities with regards to supporting students. Are they, for example, in an *enhanced role* such as a practice educator or lecturer practitioner, or are they assessors or supervisors? Consider these roles and identify any unique and shared features. Finally, think about how you will complement this skill set in your role as a supervisor and/or assessor.

There is no model answer to this activity as it is based on your own experiences.

Your critical thinking in Activity 2.1 might have resulted in you more clearly recognising the many different students in your area, each with a range of needs, strengths, expectations and concerns. Also, your colleagues, who have a part to play in supporting them, will have some overlap in their roles. Placement learning environments need to ensure that students get the best experiences possible to meet their needs while protecting the patient and the student. A large part of your role as supervisor/assessor is about making this happen.

Scenario 2.1 outlines the diverse range of students that supervisors and assessors support.

Scenario 2.1

Central 1 is a busy community clinical area that comprises a large integrated care team in a diverse city. There is a large number of staff working in Central 1 and a wide range of students who have varying lengths of placements. Central 1 works closely with the medical and mental health wards and students from these areas often visit for short periods of time in order to experience community and integrated working.

Jethro is a registered nurse and experienced supervisor. He is responsible for ensuring Central 1 is an effective environment for all students. He has worked there for a number of years and has a good working relationship with the two universities from which students usually come. Recently, he has noticed that the student population is more diverse, both in demographic makeup and the course or study they are undertaking. His colleagues have told him that they are a little confused by the wide range of students and at times are unclear as to how best support them.

The above scenario is typical of many busy clinical areas and this places increased pressure on staff to effectively support students, including those with a disability. Hopefully, students who have a disability will have disclosed this and any requirements or adjustments for placement learning should be clearly recorded and shared with the placement area. Although there is very little literature about how to best support student nurses with a disability on placement, the general consensus is that these students are more likely to succeed on placement if they disclose what requirements or adjustments they need (Tee et al., 2010). Although some students may be reluctant to do this, it is important that the benefits are outlined to them and support offered should they experience problems receiving any adjustments or support on placement. The report of the investigation carried out by the Disability Rights Commission into students of registrable professions including nursing, proposes a number of recommendations to regulatory bodies, universities, employers and occupational health services. These include research into the support and reasonable adjustments these students receive and monitoring their progress and attainment (Disability Rights Commission, 1985).

The following sections in this chapter will help you to identify effective strategies for creating and maintaining an effective learning environment while valuing learning and creating opportunities for collaboration.

Creating and maintaining a safe learning environment

This section focuses on how you as a supervisor/assessor can create and maintain a safe and effective learning environment for students. A well planned induction can have a huge impact on student experience. Factors such as receiving timely information prior to the start of placement, being welcomed by the team and having *bite-size* clear activities and objectives are very important to students during the first couple of weeks on a new placement. In Activity 2.2 we look at how Jethro can support a range of students, including those who are at the beginning of their placement.

Activity 2.2   Critical thinking

Saskia is a second-year student Specialist Community Public Health Nurse (SCPHN). She is confident and highly motivated. This is her first week on Central 1. Devlin is a third-year student nurse. He has had a community placement before and is familiar with the environment; he thinks it is the area he wishes to work in when he qualifies. He has been on Central 1 five weeks. Rhian is a first-year Trainee Nurse Associate (TNA). She is on her first placement, although she worked as a healthcare support worker for ten years on a medical ward. She is nervous about working in the community and is anxious she receives enough supervision.

How can Jethro create and maintain an environment that meets the needs of this diverse range of students? What are the *essentials* he needs to put in place for this to happen? You may wish to list five to ten *essentials* for Jethro to implement on Central 1.

There is a model answer at the end of this chapter.

As highlighted in Activity 2.2, the clinical placement must be adaptable in order to meet students' needs. Learners will be at varying levels of experience and expertise and will have a range of proficiencies to meet. The placement should offer learning opportunities for all, and one way of achieving this is to create peer-to-peer learning opportunities. This is where students work together on a problem or scenario to resolve issues and create solutions. For example, a supervisor may be supporting a number of students during a busy shift. The supervisor can present real-life scenarios and assign specific roles and responsibilities both to individual students and to them as a team. In this way they are able to meet their individual proficiencies and learn from each other through practising team working and communication skills. Let's consider this further in Scenario 2.2.

Scenario 2.2

It is Friday afternoon and a young mum presents at Central 1 complaining of feeling lethargic and with a rash to her face and neck. She is accompanied by her two children aged 4 years and 12 months. The children's cheeks are also red and the younger one appears drowsy. The practice supervisor, Jethro, decides to involve the students in the care of this family. He spends time with them asking what they think needs to be done and to prioritise any interventions. He asks them to make a note about their decisions and the rationale for their choices. He then gets them to share this with each other and then to agree, as a group, how to care for the family. Jethro reviews their plan and makes any necessary amendments, informing the group what he has done and why. He points them to a couple of resources they can access to deepen their knowledge in these areas. Next, they agree who will undertake which activities and he arranges for them to feed back later in the day. As part of this they will provide feedback to each other about their performance and what they learnt, advising them to use a reflective model. Jethro is aware that there is a range of competence and experience in the group and also how much supervision each requires, and he makes sure that he or a colleague is available to support them.

This scenario highlights the fact that students are a fantastic resource as they can support each other and also develop their competence through team working. Involving students in peer-to-peer learning also more closely replicates the *real* world, where much care is delivered in a team environment with different professionals involved. It is also an effective and efficient way to support a diverse range of students. Learners report that they learn significant amounts from their peers when in placement (McDonough, 2016). This type of learning is often referred to as problem-based learning and it has been found to be a highly effective strategy in nurse education, especially when applied to the clinical context (Shin and Kim, 2013).

Patient safety

Ensuring that a learning environment promotes patient safety is essential to a good learning experience. In this section we will look at three areas of patient safety: human factors, consent and duty of candour. We begin with human factors.

Human factors is the study of human interactions with other elements to develop quality and safety mechanisms. It stems from aviation and engineering settings, but is widely used in healthcare and healthcare education. Human factors are those things that affect an individual's performance and as a result have an impact on patient safety. It focuses on the micro and the macro factors including person-to-person interactions, decision-making and creating safe environments in which to work. A human factors approach is key to safer healthcare as its focus is on improving practice in order to avoid mistakes and near misses (Fawcett and Rhynas, 2014). Organisations and placement areas have a role to play in promoting human factors as they give *permission* to be open about near misses and mistakes, thereby promoting a learning culture which is essential to patent safety (RCN, no date). Human factors are seen as essential to healthcare to such an extent that the NMC has embedded human factors into the new standards of proficiency for registered nurses so that all students wishing to register with the NMC must achieve this proficiency. The NMC defines human factors as *the environmental, organisational and job factors, and human and individual characteristics, which influence behaviour at work in a way which can affect health and safety* (NMC, 2018a, p39). It is well recognised that patient safety is *everybody's business* as decisions are rarely made in a **uni-professional vacuum**. Therefore, to really improve patient safety, and understand the complex human factors that are at play in the healthcare environment, education and training needs to be coordinated and delivered interprofessionally (RCN, no date).

A human factors approach to patient safety starts with an understanding of the things that support or hinder the way we work. Students who are new to your clinical environment can be a fantastic resource as they will notice things that you may not be aware of. In many ways they can be a *barometer* of patient safety. As a supervisor/assessor you can improve patient safety by seeking their feedback and looking for ways to improve. Also, they should be involved in learning from near misses and mistakes. Often, students are excluded from these discussions but including them will not only enhance their own learning (and therefore protect future patients) but will also enhance the culture and practice of your clinical area.

Students, no matter where they are in their learning journey, will be familiar with the importance of reflecting on practice. In your role as supervisor/assessor you can support them to develop this to enhance patient safety. A study undertaken in 2016 in Sweden found that using a three-step model of reflection following simulated learning enhanced students' learning and attitudes (Lestander et al., 2016). The model included written and verbal reflections where steps 1 and 3 are written reflections and step 2 is a verbal group reflection. The findings from the study demonstrated an increased commitment to patient safety. One participant reported the value of making a mistake in the simulated scenario. She thought the learning would stay with her and as a result help her prepare for future situations. The new pre-registration standards (NMC, 2018a) place more emphasis on the value of simulation in student learning. We have identified that simulation is a valuable and authentic learning mode which can occur in AEI or practice areas. Activity 2.3 helps you to consider the opportunities for simulation in your practice area.

Activity 2.3   Decision-making

Review your student's practice assessment documents and their learning goals for the placement. Make a list of the proficiencies that might best be met by simulated learning activities. This may because there is little or no opportunity to practise them in *real life* or the learning may be enhanced through simulation, for example creating a patient safety scenario for the students to work on together. Try to identify which proficiencies might be best achieved via simulated learning. You may wish to view the evidence base for this and look for policies and practice in your workplace. Identify one or two from this list. We suggest you start with something that might be easy to accomplish and not requiring too much resource: a win–win! Now think about how you will deliver this learning activity: Where? When? How? Who? What resources are required? Are there any obstacles? Once you have delivered the activity reflect back on what went well and what could be done differently and share this learning with colleagues. There may be a nurse academic, for example a link lecturer, at the AEI who could support you to deliver the activity and work on any enhancements.

There is no model answer for this activity as this is based on your own experiences.

Activity 2.3 looks at the value of human factors to patient safety. More information about simulation as a teaching method can be found in Chapter 5. This next section looks at another aspect of patient safety and its importance to maintaining a safe environment for patients and students: informed consent.

Central to managing risk is information-giving and consent-seeking. Supervisors need to demonstrate to their students how to convey often complex information, check understanding and gain consent. These are complex and subtle skills and the supervisors must make these overt to enable the student to acquire them. Prior to an interaction with a patient you should talk through with your students the information you are sharing, how you intend to share it and how you will check understanding and gain consent. Make it clear what the goals of the interaction are and how they relate to the patient's care plan. Unfortunately, some students report that the practice of consent seeking can be highly variable. This can lead to missed opportunities for engaging in patient care, especially in relation to an intimate or invasive procedure (Carson-Stevens et al., 2013). Chapter 3 discusses consent in relation to students being involved in people's care delivery, so you may wish to review this now.

Another key factor in patient safety is *duty of candour*, and this goes hand-in-hand with information giving and consent seeking. The duty of candour of healthcare professionals and organisations was introduced in 2015 following the recommendation of the 2013 Francis Inquiry (NHS Executive, 2015). It means that as nurses we must be honest and discuss with patients when things have gone wrong and have caused harm, or have the potential to do so. Healthcare professionals must also inform managers of adverse incidents and *near misses* (NMC, no date) The duty of candour extends to healthcare organisations too, which must support staff to report near misses and adverse events and make sure that there are clear mechanisms to do so. This is because organisations that support staff to speak up when things go wrong are more able to learn from mistakes and better protect patients from harm. All NHS Trusts will be required to publish a charter for openness and transparency so that staff have clear expectations of how they will be treated if they witness and report clinical errors (Glasper, 2016). You may wish to look at the NMC's guidance on escalating concerns (NMC, 2017c). Also familiarise yourself with your organisation's information about duty of candour and the related processes to be followed and share these with students.

Students need to be empowered to act if they witness behaviours and practice that are harmful. Role models are powerful in this context. Standard 3.1 of the NMC (2018d) *Standards Framework for Nursing and Midwifery Education* and *Part 2: Standards for Student Supervision and Assessment* states: *practice supervisors serve as role models for safe and effective practice in line with their code of conduct.* Your students will be observing how you behave in situations that are not in a patient's best interest and this may affect their behaviours and decision-making when faced with a similar scenario (Chapter 3 discusses escalation of concerns in more detail). A recent study found that practice-based mentors who are able to role model professional attributes appear to be crucial in the development of professional attributes and behaviours in student nurses (Felstead and Springett, 2016). There is a detailed section on role modelling in Chapter 5.

Valuing the learning environment and building a learning culture

Your clinical area is more than a place in which to care for patients; it is also a learning environment – an active classroom if you like. As a supervisor or assessor you are instrumental in creating this learning space. This next section helps you to do this by looking at how to build a learning culture, to ensure that placements are inclusive of all students and, of course, make use of the evidence and best practice.

A learning environment can be difficult to define and there are a number of definitions. The Royal College of Nursing describes a practice placement as a place where learning opportunities are available for students to undertake practice under the supervision of a range of practitioners in the team. It is the environment where students meet and develop therapeutic relationships with a range of service users and their carers.

The NMC (2018b, p5) describes effective practice learning as one where:

> All students are provided with safe, effective and inclusive learning experiences. Each learning environment has the governance and resources needed to deliver education and training. Students actively participate in their own education, learning from a range of people across a variety of settings.

There are 11 standards outlining how this can be achieved (NMC, 2018b).

The Placements in Focus project (ENB, 2001) produced a practice placement checklist to highlight areas of strength and those requiring improvement. This ranged from a placement area's philosophy down to whether a resource area is available to students. The checklist has a qualitative approach and asks staff to consider if care is based on best evidence and if interpersonal and practice skills are fostered through teaching and learning methods. We often focus more heavily on the practical aspects of placement areas and don't pay adequate attention to the culture and philosophy and how these impinge on learning. Although the checklist was written in 2001, it is still relevant and useful in helping to build a learning culture. More details can be found in the further reading section at the end of this chapter.

Many studies have looked at the culture of practice learning environments to determine the factors that help and hinder learning. A list of these factors is displayed in Table 2.1 (Lewin, 2007; Chuan and Barnett, 2012).

Factors that support learning	Factors that inhibit learning
Feeling welcomed	Students having to *compete* for learning opportunities
Friendly staff	Being delegated menial tasks that do not challenge
Supervisors who are familiar with students' course and learning outcomes	The placement being too busy to enable students adequate opportunity to practice
Supervision from registered staff	Staff not interested in supervising students
Diverse learning experiences	Unfriendly staff
Peer support and learning from other students	Students who are not actively engaged in their learning

Table 2.1 Factors that influence student learning on placement

You will see from studying Table 2.1 that if students feel welcomed by friendly, approachable staff it has a positive impact on their learning. Interestingly, ward staff often perceive their clinical area to be friendlier compared to students' perceptions. This could be for a number of reasons including their familiarity with the ward and staff and also increased confidence. Students report that rotating around clinical areas is stressful as they feel they have to 'fit in' to each new area. The learning from this is that we need to be very aware of how we welcome students onto our clinical area to help them feel supported.

It would seem that staff attitudes and behaviour exert a significant influence on the learning environment and how it is perceived by students. It is, of course, difficult to separate out staff behaviours from other aspects of the learning environment. However, there are a number of other factors that influence the learning environment, which include:

- teaching and learning activities that place the students as passive recipients;
- a focus on factual recall, which can be intimidating to students and also stifle problem solving;
- vague objectives that are confusing to students and result in time being spent trying to navigate these rather than learning;
- placement areas that do not optimise the potential for **interprofessional learning** (the benefits of which are outlined in Chapter 3).

Table 2.1 outlines a number of practical issues that have a negative effect on learning; one of the most commonly cited is students feeling that they are competing for learning opportunities and tasks to enable them to meet proficiencies. This can be related to poor planning, where learning opportunities are ad hoc and increase the sense of competitiveness and anxiety in students. However, there are some quick fixes and longer-term solutions that can address these. Examples of these are:

- Involve a group of students in a discussion following an event or intervention. This is particularly useful when it would have been unfeasible for all students to be involved in the actual event. The post event discussion and analysis can be an equally powerful learning experience.
- Ensure that you and the student are clear what their objectives are for the whole placement, each week and each shift and review these regularly.
- Plan learning opportunities with the student. Students can co-construct their learning opportunities with you. Identify the opportunities available and work with your team to maximise student involvement.
- Empower students to ask questions, make suggestions and give feedback.
- Make overt connections between theory and practice learning, e.g. *You have learnt about risk factors in relation to falls, we are now going to assess patient X to determine their risk. What are the key areas we should cover and which assessment tools should we consider using?*
- Engage all staff in student learning, including managers and senior staff. Try to create a structured learning programme into which staff from a range of professions provide input.

Activity 2.4 is your opportunity to look at the strengths and limitations of your practice area.

Activity 2.4   Leadership and management

Using the information in this chapter complete a SWOT (Strengths, Weaknesses, Opportunities, Threats) analysis of your clinical learning environment. Once you have completed the SWOT analysis identify two actions you wish to adopt in the short term.

Strengths (often internal to your organisation)	Weaknesses (often internal to your organisation)
These may be cultural such as attitudes and motivations of your colleagues	*These may be related to resources or levels of expertise and experience*
Opportunities (often external to your organisation)	Threats (often external to your organisation)
These may include the strength of the relationships with the AEI	*These could include changes or requirements imposed by external bodies or organisations*

There is no model answer for this activity as it is based on your own clinical area.

The earlier sections covered in this chapter have enabled us to consider practice learning environments in their widest sense. This next section looks at one type of learning which is often associated with practice learning: work-based learning.

Work-based learning

As stated earlier, there are now more diverse roles and routes into healthcare than ever before. Apprenticeships are a popular option in healthcare as they require less time away from the workplace as they are based around a work-based learning (WBL) approach. There are many definitions of WBL, but the following sums it up succinctly: learning for work, learning at work, learning from work (Burton and Jackson, 2003). WBL builds on **experiential learning** theory, which is described in Chapter 4. Apprentices will spend most of their time in the workplace, with a requirement to engage in at least 20 per cent *off the job training*. This is a different approach to the standard degree route to nurse education. Many apprentices may be established employees, possibly nursing assistants etc., so while they may be familiar with the clinical area and colleagues they will need to adopt a new role and acquire skills and knowledge to meet proficiencies. Supervisors need to support students to transition into this role and ensure that their time for learning is not eroded with work responsibilities and tasks (Rosser, 2017). The ability to facilitate learning on the job and apply practice experience to theory is essential when supporting this type of student.

Learning organisations

As a result of completing Activity 2.4. you may have identified that some strengths and threats may be exerted by your organisation (hospital, Trust etc.). These may include how your organisation enables or hinders your attempts to build a learning culture. The introduction of the duty of candour should create a more open and transparent approach to learning and a move away from a blame culture. There is more of an acceptance that people do make mistakes and by being open and reflecting on them creates a culture of learning and patient safety (Glasper, 2016). However, learning organisations go beyond this and are not interested in avoidance of harm or maintenance of a steady state. Instead, they are open to system-wide changes that bring about transformed care. Features of learning organisations include a focus on team learning and capability as opposed to individual learning. This team learning approach needs to transcend artificial boundaries and networks, such as department and clinical specialities, and look to the whole organisation. Challenging people's assumptions about the world, including healthcare, allows greater learning to take place and promotes innovation. Underneath all of this is a shared vision, one that people can make sense of and buy into. Lastly, one vital yet often overlooked feature of an organisation that wants to be a 'learning organisation' is the celebration of success and valuing achievements (Davies and Nutley, 2000).

Learning for all

When creating a learning environment, it is essential that it meets the needs of a diverse range of students and is inclusive with equity of opportunity. Chapter 5 looks at these issues in detail. When you are preparing to welcome students to your clinical area, it is recommended that you consider what their needs might be and how you can adjust your behaviours, expectations and the learning environment to accommodate them.

The evidence-informed supervisor/assessor

Just as your practice as a registered nurse is informed by the evidence base, so should your practice as a supervisor/assessor. This does not only relate to demonstrating the best practice to students and supervising them to achieve this for themselves, but also how you deliver best practice in your role of supervisor/assessor.

This book includes much around the evidence base on coaching, supervising, teaching and assessment. Therefore, reading this book and completing the activities in it means that you are engaging in evidence-based supervision and assessment. However, what about opportunities to move beyond this and improve your own practice? By this, we mean creating and disseminating evidence and best practice. As a supervisor/assessor of students you are in a perfect position to do this. This is because almost all of the students you support will be enrolled on an AEI course, be that a nursing degree or other. Academic colleagues will be supporting you and your colleagues to enable you to best support the students while out on placement. This is your opportunity to engage in collaborations with these staff. Many staff at the AEI will be engaged in scholarly activity. This may include undertaking research, postgraduate or doctoral study, presenting at conferences and writing articles and books. Some of this scholarly activity will be focused on practice-based learning and how this can be improved. Your experience as a supervisor/assessor is invaluable and offers you the opportunity to collaborate. This may be in a number of ways:

- being a participant in a research project, e.g. your experiences of being a supervisor;
- implementing the recommendations of a research project into your clinical area – such as a new model for supporting students in practice;
- attending as a guest lecturer – to talk about supervising and assessing in practice;
- co-authoring a journal article with a colleague from the AEI – this may be about joint working;
- collaborating on a service improvement project – such as patient involvement in student assessment and feedback.

Chapter 8 includes more detail on your continuing professional development as a supervisor/assessor. While you are developing your confidence and skill as a supervisor/assessor you may wish to think about how you can collaborative and engage in evidence-based practice in relation to supervising and assessing and Activity 2.5 helps you start this process.

Activity 2.5 Evidence-based research

This is your opportunity for some *blue-sky* thinking. Imagine you are about to engage in some scholarly activity on the area of supporting students in practice. You are going to collaborate with a lecturer from your local AEI. What would you suggest you collaborate on? Look at the list of scholarly activities above to help you. Now think about topic areas. What are you particularly interested in? Which areas do you think there are gaps in our knowledge and understanding? What do you think people might like to read or hear about?

Once you have done some free thinking and scribbled down your ideas start to narrow them down to two or three. Now do the final step, which is to choose one. You might do this rationally and list strengths, limitations and feasibility etc., or you might go with your *gut* feeling. Now that you have chosen one, why not put together a very brief proposal outlining what the

(Continued)

(Continued)

activity is, any background literature and how the scholarly activity might help develop understanding of that area. Ask a colleague who you trust to look at it and then make any amendments you wish to. Now for the hard bit! Contact your AEI link person and ask if you can talk through an idea you have for some scholarly activity.

There is no model answer for this activity as it is based on your own reflections.

Chapter summary

This chapter has identified the key components of a positive learning environment and has outlined the supervisor and assessor roles in preserving safety. The diverse range of students and modes of study means that there is greater complexity for practice supervisors and assessors. However, this also increases the opportunities for interprofessional and work-based learning, both of which are seen as valuable in the acquisition of competence in healthcare education and delivery.

Activity answers

Activity 2.2: Critical thinking (p30)

Jethro needs to make every student feel welcome and ensure that there are learning opportunities for all. Although the team may be more experienced and familiar with supporting student nurses, they need to attend to the needs of all students such as Saskia and Rhian. Jethro could do lots of things but here are some suggestions:

- Devise a welcome pack to all students that is not profession specific nor heavily student nurse focused.
- Create a list of all the learning opportunities, including visits and specialist practitioners, and identify which students they may be most relevant to.
- Invite the link academics from the universities to visit to brief the staff on all of the types of students, their programmes and any unique needs (such as end-point assessment).
- Provide an outline from each type of student detailing the programme they are on and what they hope to get from the placement.
- Schedule an update session familiarising the staff with the proficiencies and practice assessment documentation.
- Create an opportunity for frequently asked questions (FAQs), either face to face, online or in a student file.
- Ask supervisors who have supported these types of students to talk about their experiences and offer tips.

- Create opportunities for interprofessional learning to enable students and colleagues to learn *with, from and about each other.*
- Develop a book, a little like a hotel guests' comments book, where past students can leave comments about their experience and the opportunities they found useful and they would recommend.

Further reading

English National Board for Nursing, Midwifery and Health Visiting and Department of Health (2001) *Placements in Focus.* Guidance for education in practice and healthcare professions. This guidance was developed as a result of work undertaken to both increase the placement capacity and ensure quality and consistency of placement learning. It includes a useful checklist to help with the planning, provision and evaluation of practice placement learning.

Royal College of Nursing (2017a) toolkit titled: *Helping Students Get the Best from Their Practice Placements: A Royal College of Nursing Toolkit.* It is available from the RCN website. Although it is written for students, it is a really useful toolkit that would be good reading for novice practice supervisors. The document was published in 2017 and is due for review in 2020 so it does not align to the new NMC standards. However, much of the content is still highly relevant. It's the type of document you can easily dip in and out of.

NHS Employers (2014) *What Makes a Good Placement?* This resource contains case studies from NHS Trust placement areas that were shortlisted for Student Nursing Times Awards. It is mapped against the 6Cs and identifies areas of good practice. You might find it gives you some good ideas about further developing your learning environment. **www.nhsemployers.org/case-studies-and-resources/2014/08/what-makes-a-good-student-placement**

Chapter 3 Educational governance and quality

Standards Framework for Nursing and Midwifery Education. Part 1 of Realising Professionalism: Standards for Education and Training (NMC, 2018d)

This chapter will address the standards in heading **2: Educational governance and quality.**

2.1 There are effective governance systems that ensure compliance with all legal, regulatory, professional and educational requirements, differentiating where appropriate between the devolved legislatures of the United Kingdom, with clear lines of responsibility and accountability for meeting those requirements and responding when standards are not met, in all learning environments.

2.2 All learning environments optimise safety and quality, taking account of the diverse needs of, and working in partnership with, service users, students and all other stakeholders.

The Code: Professional Standards of Practice and Behaviour for Nurses and Midwives (NMC, 2015)

This chapter most closely aligns with the following professional standards.

Prioritise people

3.4 act as an advocate for the vulnerable, challenging poor practice and discriminatory attitudes and behaviour relating to their care.

Practise effectively

6.1 make sure that any information or advice given is evidence based, including information relating to using any healthcare products or services.

6.2 maintain the knowledge and skills you need for safe and effective practice.

8.4 work with colleagues to evaluate the quality of your work and that of the team.

8.5 work with colleagues to preserve the safety of those receiving care.

8.6 share information to identify and reduce risk.

8.7 be supportive of colleagues who are encountering health or performance problems. However, this support must never compromise or be at the expense of patient or public safety.

9.4 support students' and colleagues' learning to help them develop their professional competence and confidence.

11.2 make sure that everyone you delegate tasks to is adequately supervised and supported so they can provide safe and compassionate care.

Preserve safety

16.4 acknowledge and act on all concerns raised to you, investigating, escalating or dealing with those concerns where it is appropriate for you to do so.

16.5 not obstruct, intimidate, victimise or in any way hinder a colleague, member of staff, person you care for or member of the public who wants to raise a concern.

16.6 protect anyone you have management responsibility for from any harm, detriment, victimisation or unwarranted treatment after a concern is raised.

Promote professionalism and trust

20.3 be aware at all times of how your behaviour can affect and influence the behaviour of other people.

20.8 act as a role model of professional behaviour for students and newly qualified nurses and midwives to aspire to.

23.1 cooperate with any audits of training records, registration records or other relevant audits that we may want to carry out to make sure you are still fit to practise.

25.2 support any staff you may be responsible for to follow the Code at all times. They must have the knowledge, skills and competence for safe practice; and understand how to raise any concerns linked to any circumstances where the Code has, or could be, broken.

Chapter aims

After reading this chapter, you will be clear on the roles and responsibilities of Approved Education Institutions (AEIs) and practice partners on ensuring educational governance and quality in:

- recruitment and selection;
- practice placement environment and learning opportunities;
- managing fitness to practise issues;
- managing failing students.

Introduction

Educational governance and quality is about ensuring that there are processes and practices in place to protect the public and ensure students have safe and effective environments in which to learn. We introduce Jasper in the chapter scenario who is a student who enjoys using social media. This chapter focuses on the practice setting, as it is the practice setting that is most relevant to you and your role as practice supervisor and practice assessor. The chapter starts with student recruitment and selection processes then moves on to preparation for placement, including students requiring reasonable adjustments. We then look at external factors such as policy and regulation and consider what supervisors and assessors need to do to ensure a safe and effective environment and experience for students. The chapter concludes by focusing on professional behaviour and fitness to practise.

The responsibility for ensuring educational governance and quality span the **Approved Education Institution** (AEI – which is usually a university) and the practice settings (NMC, 2018d). Partnership working is essential to ensure this happens. Supervisors, practice and academic assessors all have a role to play and need to work closely and know who to go to for support. Scenario 3.1 introduces you to Jasper to whom we will refer throughout this chapter.

Scenario 3.1

Jasper is a first-year student nurse who has recently started his placement experience in a dementia unit. He is an avid user of social media and has been since starting his course. He very much appreciates the immediacy it affords and that important discussions can be aired in a rapid format and with huge reach. Many of the lecturers at his university use social media to share good practice and engage in discussions about nursing. He is a follower of many national nurse leaders. He has a significant online presence and often talks about how much value he gets from using Twitter as a student nurse. Most of the staff on the dementia unit don't use social media, although a couple of colleagues use it on a personal basis to keep up with friends. His enthusiasm motivates some of the team to start using social media and they now follow him on Twitter.

As we can see in Scenario 3.1, many student nurses are confident in using social media and believe it has value for progressing the nursing profession. However, not all registrants are comfortable using it and some may be suspicious of its relevance to the profession.

Concerns have been highlighted relating to the effectiveness of support for students in practice settings. These concerns are evidenced in the reports from the Shape of Caring review (Willis, 2015) and the RCN Mentorship Project (RCN, 2016b). These documents have been instrumental in the development of the NMC educational framework (2018b and 2018d) on which this book based.

The following are the key recommendations from the Willis Commission (2012).

Quality with Compassion: The future of nurse education Theme 3: Learning to nurse. (Please note, the term mentor is used throughout the document as its publication preceded the NMC educational framework.)

1. The quality of many practice learning experiences urgently needs improvement. Learning to care in real-life settings lies at the heart of patient-centred education and learning to be a nurse.

2. The NMC standards must be fully implemented through active partnerships between NHS education and training boards at national and local levels, employers and universities, to ensure the quality of nursing education, and use and share existing tools and standards.

3. Managers, mentors, practice education facilitators and academic staff must work together to help students relate theory to practice. Close, effective collaboration between universities and practice settings should be enhanced through joint appointments.

4. Employers and universities must together identify positive practice environments in a wide range of settings. Many more placements must be made available in community settings, including medical general practice. The absence of funding to higher education institutions (HEIs) to support nursing students' practical learning experiences must be addressed.

5. Employers must ensure mentors have dedicated time for mentorship, while universities should play their full part in training and updating mentors. Mentors must be selected for their knowledge, skills and motivation; adequately prepared; well supported; and valued, with a recognised status.

6. Practical learning must be underpinned with relevant knowledge from clinical and social science disciplines. All students should be aware of the growing evidence base on good nursing practice. Graduate nurses, as future leaders of clinical teams, should understand how to evaluate, utilise and conduct research, and act on evidence to improve the quality of care.

Activity 3.1   Evidence-based practice and research

After reading the recommendations from the Willis Commission (2012), identify any learning points relating to your developing supervisor/assessor role and agree one activity you can complete to address these.

There is no model answer for this activity as the activity is based on your own research and individual learning needs.

As a result of a range of evidence and documents, including the Willis report (2012), the education and governance of nurse education has been overhauled and this is reflected in the new NMC education framework (2018b, 2018d). There are two stand-ards that are part of education and governance – these are: *governance and accountability* and *safety and quality assurance.* Practice supervisor and assessor roles are at the heart of these standards. We will consider governance and accountability first.

Governance and accountability are concerned with ensuring processes are in place to ensure learners are both suitable for practice and are placed in safe environments that offer them the opportunities and support they require to achieve proficiencies. This can be broken down to the following areas:

- recruitment and selection;
- local governance processes and orientating the student to these;
- data sharing;
- failing students.

Recruitment and selection – although it is the AEIs that are responsible for recruiting students, practice partners have a part to play in strengthening this. Selection processes that involve practice partners are more robust, ensuring the selection of the most appropriate students and support partnership working. AEIs will often contact prac-tice areas to request support for recruitment events. Taking part in these events can strengthen your skill set. As well as assessing learners' suitability to engage in a profes-sional programme there is also the need to ensure students meet the requirements set by the NMC, namely being of *good health and character* and that they have disclosed any criminal convictions and cautions. Criminal convictions and health conditions do not necessarily preclude students from commencing an NMC approved programme, but it is of paramount importance that these are disclosed when requested to do so.

Some students may have relevant knowledge and skills from previous learning, for example transferring between AEIs or returning to study after a significant break. These students should have the opportunity for this to be taken into account and possi-bly used to reduce the length of study. This is usually referred to as **recognition of prior learning** (RPL) and any claims for this need to meet the NMC and AEI standards and regulations.

Recruitment should be 'values-based' so as to attract and select students whose indi-vidual values and behaviours align with the values of the NHS Constitution (NHS England, 2015), outlined in Table 3.1. Recruitment and selection should assess these aptitudes and skills so that the students who are selected hold the right values to support effective team working in order to deliver excellent patient care and expe-rience (HEE, 2016). There has been an increased focus on the values held by the NHS workforce, partly as a result of the Mid Staffordshire NHS Foundation Trust Public Inquiry (Francis, 2013) which highlighted the vital role of the workforce in providing high-quality and safe healthcare. Getting involved in recruitment and

Value	Description
Working together for patients	Patients come first; patients, families, carers, communities should be involved in care design and delivery. NHS staff and organisations should speak up when things go wrong.
Respect and dignity	Every person is valued (patients, families, carers or staff) – as an individual. Their views and experiences are taken seriously. Staff are honest and open about what can and cannot be done.
Commitment to quality of care	Insist on quality and getting the basics of quality of care right every time. Feedback is welcomed and acted on to improve care.
Compassion	Compassion and kindness is central. This is active and not reactive.
Improving lives	The NHS and its staff aim to improve health and wellbeing. Excellence and professionalism is nurtured and celebrated. Everyone has a part to play in making ourselves, patients and communities healthier.
Everyone counts	Resources are maximised for the benefit of the whole community. No one (individual or communities) is excluded or discriminated against.

Table 3.1 NHS Constitution values

selection events can not only familiarise you with the whole range of expectations placed on students but you can also help shape the future workforce. Activity 3.2 will help you do this in your area.

Activity 3.2   Team working

Get in touch with your link lecturer (academic contact from your students' AEI) and volunteer to take part in any upcoming recruitment and selection events. You could also discuss the possibility of delivering a session to first-year students around preparation for practice placement. Your knowledge and experience will be invaluable to students, who evaluate these sessions highly, and also to you as a developing practice supervisor/assessor. This will also provide you with good evidence for your appraisal/personal development review and your NMC revalidation (NMC, 2017a). Once you have completed the recruitment event or teaching session, complete a reflective account using the NMC revalidation template (available on the NMC website).

There is no model answer to this activity as it is based on your own research.

Having explored recruitment and selection, we now turn our attention to students with extra needs. Students may start the programme with a known disability that may have an impact on their learning. If this is the case, the university should provide them with an assessment of their needs and any support or **reasonable adjustments** to enable them to be successful in their learning (Tee et al., 2010). However, students may develop a disability such as a mental health problem or have one assessed while undertaking the programme, most commonly dyslexia. These students may need a period of adjustment in coming to terms with this and should be given all the support required to help them. They may need to have more time to complete tasks or have other adjustments put in place such as set breaks or the opportunity to attend appointments with a range of staff such as counsellors or occupational health services (Griffiths et al., 2010). Universities have specialist services and resources for students with disabilities and students may come to your practice area with a learning contract. Although universities have established services and processes these may not be as readily available in the practice setting. Your role here is to be clear on what the student's needs are, the support they require and then facilitate this. You can contact the link lecturer also if you are unsure how to support a student with a learning contract. Students may not wish or need to disclose any details of their disability, and it is your responsibility as supervisor/assessor to protect their privacy and ensure others act respectfully and confidentially.

Local governance processes – each placement area will have local governance processes. It is important that as supervisor/assessor you orientate students to these, paying particular attention to corporate and information governance policies and procedures. It is good practice to make available any information that is relevant to the students prior to commencing the placement (e.g. dress code and uniform policy). Students need to be familiarised with and informed about IT systems and data sharing. They also need to be informed about how to escalate concerns and the procedure for any

Activity 3.3   Leadership and management

Review the information for students in your practice area. Do you have a student handbook or file? How up to date is it? Try to look at it objectively and ask yourself how helpful it is. If you don't have one, then talk to colleagues in your workplace about creating one. You may wish to contact a colleague from the education department in your organisation to ask if there are any examples of good student handbooks or a template you can use. Don't forget to talk to the students working in your area and ask them to give feedback on the existing material or suggest what additions they might find useful. Try to avoid creating just a collection of documents. It is probably more useful to include a paragraph outlining why the information has been included, how the reader might use it and how it might help them during the placement. Students will also value links to online resources, such as learning objects and training resources.

There is no model answer for this activity as it is based on your own research.

untoward incident such as injury or assault. Completing Activity 3.3 will help you develop the related information available to students in your clinical area. Having clear and detailed information provides evidence of the support available to students, which may be reviewed during internal and external monitoring.

Data sharing – practice areas and education institutions are regularly reviewed and monitored via internal processes and external bodies including the **Quality Assurance Agency**, **Care Quality Commission** and the Nursing and Midwifery Council. The outcomes of these events may have implications for student learning and it is important you are clear about any issues identified and recommendations made. The last report from the CQC or your Trust or practice area will include a list of areas of good practice and areas to improve. General Data Protection Regulation (GDPR) came into effect in May 2018. The aim of this new legislation, which replaces the Data Protection Act, is to update and strengthen data protection regulation in the EU. The government has confirmed that Brexit will not affect the UK's compliance with GDPR as it offers best practice for handling and sharing data. This is highly relevant legislation for you as clinical practitioners but also as supervisors and/or assessors (Astrup, 2018).

Escalating concerns and failing students – of course, not every student is successful in meeting the proficiencies in practice and may fail. If this isn't something you have experienced, or haven't experienced for some time, then you may wish to familiarise yourself with the process and support available to you as a supervisor/assessor. The AEI will have clear guidance about this so get in touch with the contact person (e.g. link lecturer or academic advisor) and ask for the information. It's much easier to digest this type of information when you are not in the midst of managing a difficult situation. Vinales (2015) has created a useful algorithm that can be used by practice supervisors and assessors to support them in making decisions about competence. This step-by-step approach clearly identifies decision points for supervisors and assessors and in doing so reduces the risks of leaving it very late before any issues around student competence are escalated. Activity 3.4 touches on issues such as fitness to practise, professional behaviours and escalating concerns.

Scenario 3.2

Jasper has been tweeting about his experiences on the dementia unit and how much he is learning on the placement. He has a large number of followers and many of his tweets have been retweeted. A member of the team reads his tweets and is concerned about some of them. She thinks that some of the content makes the placement area easily identifiable and potentially breaches patient confidentiality. She speaks to Precious, Jasper's practice accessor, about the content.

Social media is used regularly by nursing and midwifery students as well as healthcare professionals, and can be a fantastic vehicle to enhance learning. There is growing literature on how the different generations (baby boomers through to Generation Z) relate uniquely to social media and this can lead to differences in opinion about its usefulness and appropriateness (Health Education England, 2015). See Chapter 4 for more information on generational differences. However, social media is regularly implicated in fitness to practise concerns. Scenario 3.2 highlights one of these issues and how Jasper's practice assessor Precious might respond. Activity 3.4 gives you the opportunity to explore further the issues identified in Scenario 3.2.

Activity 3.4   Decision-making

Consider how Precious, from Scenario 3.2, should respond to the concerns raised by her colleague about Jethro's use of Twitter. Identify three actions and make a note of these.

There is a model answer for this activity at the end of the chapter.

Although Activity 3.4 focuses on Precious, as the student's practice assessor, the responsibility for supporting students who are failing in practice is the joint responsibility of the AEI and the practice area. These students must be given opportunities to succeed, and practice and education partners must work closely to help them (see Chapter 6 for guidance on action planning in such an instance). However, if after support, a student is not competent to pass, the decision must be made to fail them (Duffy, 2003; Gainsbury, 2010). The decision that a student has passed or failed is one of the most transparent acts of accountability for the practice assessor and if the decision is that they have failed then this can be a stressful time for all involved. If you find yourself in this situation then it may be helpful to seek support from an experienced assessor or a colleague from your practice learning team to help you through this process (see Chapter 7 for more on this).

Safety and quality assurance are concerned with protecting the public and the student by ensuring safe learning environments and promoting professional behaviours. These three areas are:

- preparing and maintaining the learning environment;
- keeping up to date with the curriculum and curriculum development;
- promoting professional behaviour.

Preparing and maintaining a safe and effective learning environment – the whole of the team have a role to play in preparing and maintaining a safe and effective learning environment. Although one person may take a lead, they rely heavily on colleagues' commitment and expertise. Prior to students commencing placement, it is a requirement that there is an up-to-date placement audit. This is undertaken jointly by the practice area and the AEI. It should include details about the number and types of students who can be placed and an agreement that there are suitably prepared and supported supervisors and assessors. In addition, the practice area must be safe and offer learning opportunities to enable the student to meet the proficiencies. Students must be able to access a range of opportunities and given time and support to develop their knowledge and skills. The AEI and NMC need to be assured that the placement can achieve all of the above and the close working partnership between practice and AEI is key to making this happen. Once the audit has been agreed by both parties, then students can be placed there. Practice areas must be given information by the AEI about the start and end dates of student placements and where the students are in their programme of study. However, it is your responsibility as supervisor/assessor to prepare for the students' arrival.

Students report that it is often the little things that make a big difference to their placement experience and learning. These can be: students being informed who their supervisor/assessor is prior to commencing; being sent information about the placement; having a shift pattern for the first week or so and having a safe place to store their belongings (Hamshire et al., 2012). Activity 3.5 will help you identify what might make a difference to the students coming to your practice area.

Activity 3.5 Team working

Take a look at the information given by your practice area to students before they start their placement. Make a note of what you think needs to remain and what could be removed or added. Now think about how you induct a student to your practice area. Does this induction make them part of the team or are they sometimes treated differently? For example, where do they take a break? What's the protocol for buying drinks like tea and coffee? Where do they store their belongings? Are they invited out to social events or to join in on other informal activities such as book swaps etc.?

Once you have completed the above, consider if anything needs to be done differently to help students develop a sense of belonging and being part of the team.

There is a model answer to this activity at the end of the chapter.

It is also important that the learning environment is safe and effective throughout the whole of the student's time with you. Gaining feedback from students about the range and quality of learning opportunities and responding to issues quickly and efficiently will ensure this is more robust. It may be that exceptional circumstances arise while a student is with you, for example, an outbreak of infection, the presence of a particularly unpredictable or dangerous patient, or there are serious concerns following an inspection. You may need to consider, along with the student, AEI and practice education team, whether it is appropriate for the student to remain or whether they should move to another area for a period of time. If this is the case, then an action plan may need to be drawn up with the student that minimises the impact of this on their learning. Although these situations may not be very common, it is worth agreeing with the AEI how you best prepare for them. This would probably fall into the role of the person in your clinical area who is the named link to the AEI; or you might have a colleague identified as a learning environment manager. They may agree this process when completing the audit.

Keeping up to date on curriculum development – students should be very familiar with the content of their programme and which proficiencies they need to achieve while they are with you. It is important that you are also familiar with the programme and particularly the practice assessment documentation. One quick win is to attend update events that are usually delivered by the link lecturer from the AEI. These usually occur in the practice setting or online, and often include an overview of the programme, the practice assessment documentation and opportunities for questions and answers. In addition, there are usually digital resources available including the full training plan for each cohort of students and academic staff contact details. However, AEIs are continuously improving their education programmes and value the input and feedback from practice partners on new proposals and enhancements. In fact, it is a requirement of the NMC that practice partners have been consulted when a programme is being approved (by the NMC and AEI). This is a perfect opportunity for you to influence the education of the next generation of nurses. Your experience as a practitioner and practice supervisor/assessor is invaluable and the AEI would value your input. You may wish to express your interest to your link lecturer about getting involved in such events.

Promoting professional behaviours – one of the most influential aspects of being a practice supervisor/assessor is developing the professional behaviours of students. The NMC guide on enabling professionalism outlines the five domains of individual professionalism (NMC, 2017b). These are learning and developing continuously; being a role model for others; supporting appropriate service and care environments; enabling person-centred and evidence-informed practice; and leading professionally. These domains can be clearly articulated against your role as supervisor/assessor. Probably the most relevant is *being a role model for others*, as the values you express and how you act in a range of situations is very powerful in shaping students' own values and behaviours. Being a role model includes the following behaviours and attributes: celebrating diversity; supporting colleagues and students; celebrating success (own and others); developing people to take on leadership roles and activities; and providing constructive feedback. In addition, another powerful attribute is the ability to accept and respond to constructive feedback and be *open* to self-development. Chapter 5 has a detailed section on role modelling that you may find helpful to read before completing Activity 3.6.

Scenario 3.3

Precious reads Jasper's tweets and, after reflecting on them and discussing with another experienced practice assessor, determines that he has not breached confidentiality. However, she does think that the tweets can be a little flippant and open to misinterpretation. She feeds this back to him and he is genuinely surprised. Their conversation then turns to how difficult it can be to communicate complex information via social media. She is aware that the different generations can relate differently to social media: she is Generation X and Jasper is Z. She reflects on their discussion and decides she will take more time to demonstrate how to convey complex and sensitive information in order to make this more explicit to him. She values Jasper's courage and commitment – these are key principles of the 6Cs – and doesn't want to undermine his confidence but also thinks he needs to develop his skills around conveying complex information. Precious thinks back to one of her mentors and remembers what a brilliant role model she was and how much it made her want be a mentor; she hopes that she can also be a good role model to Jasper.

Activity 3.6 explores further how the role modeler needs to show compassionate practice and leadership to enable the student to learn from the situation.

Activity 3.6   Critical thinking

In Scenario 3.3, think about the behaviours Precious could demonstrate to Jasper. What situations and learning opportunities should she try to make available to Jasper to enable him to develop in these areas? How can she make this learning more powerful for him? Jot down your thoughts to these questions.

There is a model answer at the end of the chapter.

> ## Chapter summary
>
> ....
>
> As a result of reading this chapter and completing the activities you should be familiar with educational governance and quality and your role and responsibilities in assuring these. The Willis report highlighted both inadequacies and best practice. The subsequent NMC educational framework sets out the requirements for ensuring safe and effective learning environments. How we recruit students and prepare and maintain the learning environment are integral elements of this. The chapter also considered how students should be supported to enable them to achieve, including those requiring reasonable adjustments. The chapter concluded by considering fitness to practise and professional behaviours and the importance of the practice supervisor and assessor as role models in upholding these and ultimately protecting patients and the public.

Activity answers

Activity 3.4: Decision-making (p50)

The following answer is not exhaustive but Precious should in the first instance gather a little more evidence. She should view the content of Jasper's tweets and after viewing them make an assessment of the content and whether there are any breaches of confidentiality. Precious should get in touch with the link lecturer or other contact from the AEI and inform them of the situation and ask for information and guidance regarding using social media and make sure Jasper has a copy and understands it. She should then meet with Jasper in private and share the concerns with him. If she does not think there are any fitness to practise issues she should feed back that other colleagues have raised concerns and also advise him to carefully consider the content of his posts. If she does have issues regarding fitness to practise she should meet with the link lecturer and agree with them how to progress this. She should ask Jasper to refrain from discussing his placement experiences on social media while they are investigating the concerns. Precious should inform her colleague who raised concerns that the situation is being managed, while protecting Jasper's confidentiality, and keep Jasper updated on any developments.

Activity 3.5: Team working (p51)

The evidence suggests that there are a number of things that help students to orientate to and feel part of the team and succeed on placement (Eick et al., 2012). These include:

- acceptance in the workplace;
- feeling supported by the team;
- having a strong sense of nursing as a profession;
- opportunity to discuss and make sense of difficult experiences.

Activity 3.6: Critical thinking (p53)

The following answer is not exhaustive but Precious could allow Jasper to observe her communicating complex and sensitive information to a client or family member. An example of this might be discussing the impact on the family of a dementia diagnosis. During this consultation she should convey empathy and allow time for reflection and clarification by the family and support them should they get upset. She should offer them the opportunity to ask questions and meet with her again if they wish to. Precious should check their understanding and give written information, including support organisations to them.

Precious can make this learning opportunity more powerful to Jasper by checking his understanding of her interventions and possible rationale for these. She could use self-disclosure to increase his self-awareness, for example that she felt sad when talking to the family. She could then link this back to the tweets and how difficult it can be to communicate complex and sensitive information, especially via social media. Finally, she may suggest Jasper uses this situation as the basis of a reflective account. It is important she reassures Jasper that this is a learning opportunity, so he doesn't feel he has been chastised. This will make it more likely that he will ask for support in future, which ultimately enhances practice and protects patients.

Further reading

Are You Ready for GDPR? – essential information and a useful toolkit produced by the RCN, specifically aimed at nurses. It is helpful to refer to with regards to your responsibilities. It is available online at **www.rcn.org.uk/magazines/activate/2018/march/gdpr**.

The NMC Guidance on Using Social Media – **www.nmc.org.uk/globalassets/sitedocuments/ nmc-publications/social-media-guidance.pdf** – this helpful document applies social media use to the code and outlines best practice when engaging with social media. We suggest you signpost every student to it at the start of their placement.

NMC Enabling Professionalism – **www.nmc.org.uk/globalassets/sitedocuments/other-publications/ enabling-professionalism.pdf** – this is a great resource to help students to understand and develop professional behaviours

Useful websites

Health Education England – values based recruitment – **www.hee.nhs.uk/our-work/values-based-recruitment**. Excellent resources to support values based recruitment of students and employees.

NMC (2017) **http://revalidation.nmc.org.uk** – includes everything you need to know about the revalidation process.

Care Quality Commission – **www.cqc.org.uk** – find out more about the role and work of the CQC generally or your practice area/Trust.

Chapter 4   Student empowerment

Standards Framework for Nursing and Midwifery Education. Part 1 of Realising Professionalism: Standards for Education and Training (NMC, 2018d)

This chapter will address the standards in heading **3: Student empowerment.**

3.1 Students are provided with a variety of learning opportunities and appropriate resources, which enable them to achieve proficiencies and programme outcomes and be capable of demonstrating the professional behaviours in the NMC Code (NMC, 2015).

3.2 Students are empowered and supported to become resilient, caring, reflective and life-long learners who are capable of working in inter-professional and inter-agency teams.

The Code: Professional Standards of Practice and Behaviour for Nurses and Midwives (NMC, 2015)

This chapter most closely aligns with the following professional standards.

Practise effectively

6.2 maintain the knowledge and skills you need for safe and effective practice.

7.1 use terms that people in your care, colleagues and the public can understand.

7.2 take reasonable steps to meet people's language and communication needs, providing, wherever possible, assistance to those who need help to communicate their own or other people's needs.

7.3 use a range of verbal and non-verbal communication methods, and consider cultural sensitivities, to better understand and respond to people's personal and health needs.

7.4 Check people's understanding from time to time to keep misunderstanding or mistakes to a minimum.

8.2   maintain effective communication with colleagues.

9.3   deal with differences of professional opinion with colleagues by discussion and informed debate, respecting their views and opinions and behaving in a professional way at all times.

9.4   support students' and colleagues' learning to help them develop their professional competence and confidence.

11.1 only delegate tasks and duties that are within the other person's scope of competence, making sure that they fully understand your instructions.

11.2 make sure that everyone you delegate tasks to is adequately supervised and supported so they can provide safe and compassionate care.

11.3 confirm that the outcome of any task you have delegated to someone else meets the required standard.

Promote professionalism and trust

20.7 make sure you do not express your personal beliefs (including political, religious or moral beliefs) to people in an inappropriate way.

20.8 act as a role model of professional behaviour for students and newly qualified nurses and midwives to aspire to.

Chapter aims

After reading this chapter, you will be able to:

- understand what is meant by the terms student empowerment and autonomy;
- develop an understanding of key learning theories and styles;
- articulate the benefits to students of peer learning and interprofessional learning;
- reflect upon the impact of generational differences on learning preferences for students.

Introduction

This chapter starts by considering student empowerment as a prerequisite for effective learning and the importance of learning **autonomy**. We then consider the different approaches put forward by educational theorists to help us better understand how learning occurs. We identify different learning styles and preferences. The activities will help us to think about the relevance of these for different students we are working with. During this chapter we are introduced to Sumatra who is a practice supervisor working with a number of students, and she has been helping them to develop a clinical skill. We meet her as she is reflecting upon the challenges that one of her students posed during the session, and she is thinking about the complexities involved in the process of learning. Peer and interprofessional learning are then introduced, and the relevance and some benefits of these approaches for students are identified. The chapter concludes by considering the implications of generational differences on students' learning.

Empowerment and learner autonomy

Empowerment and autonomy are terms that are often used together, sometimes interchangeably, and have become central components of health policy in relation to patient/client/service user care. But what do these terms mean when applied to learning and students? Learner autonomy describes self-directed and independent learning where the student takes responsibility for their own learning requirements. Empowerment is a process required to enable the student to become an autonomous learner, and continues to develop as they become increasingly independent (Allen, 2010). This is critical in becoming a lifelong learner, which is a requirement for our professional registration.

For students to be empowered learners, they need to: have access to a range of learning opportunities; have a say in shaping and directing opportunities and have a choice for meaningful and purposeful engagement. Many educational theorists would argue that the most powerful and deep learning only occurs through learner autonomy. For those of us supporting learning, we can have a huge impact on leading students to a more empowered state.

Here are some examples of how to support learner autonomy and empowerment with your students:

- **Create** a supervisory relationship with your student with an emphasis on student-initiated question asking, rather than you asking all the questions. Ensure your student has access to yourself, colleagues and other resources to help with answering their questions.
- **Ask** the student to talk about what they already know and skills they have gained. Encourage them to highlight areas they need to focus on during this learning opportunity. This might be identifying any gaps they have in their repertoire of skills or developing their practice around particular theory they have recently been introduced to.
- **Actively introduce and network** the student with other students, colleagues, resources who will be helpful in their learning journey.

- **Plan** activities that help the student to impact the wider environment they are working in. For example, handing over their care interventions to others, presenting case histories to others, etc.
- **Emphasise** the uniqueness of the student's experiences and learning journey. Even previous negative experiences the student may disclose can be repackaged as learning opportunities.
- Ensure the **language** you use is appropriate for the student to be able to participate in relevant conversations. Be mindful of jargon and acronyms that are commonplace in your area, but might be unfamiliar to any newcomers.
- **Value** what your student has to say. Positively encourage participation in conversations you are having involving care that your student is involved with. Create an atmosphere of mutual respect. Talking *at* the student, ignoring their thoughts and ideas, will disempower.
- If a student's ideas and thoughts don't correspond with yours or the necessary standards for practice, don't simply dismiss them. Instead, **encourage** the student to think about alternative ideas, introducing any relevant evidence, policy, guidelines supporting these. Provide time to discuss these developing ideas and thoughts.

Many of these examples are ideally best started in the induction stage when you first meet with your student. Induction is discussed in more detail in Chapter 2.

Scenario 4.1

Sumatra is a practice supervisor and earlier this week she was working with a number of students from different courses and year groups who have just started placements in her practice area. In particular, she was teaching them about intravenous infusions. Sumatra had developed a session on anatomy with handouts, as well as facilitating a practical demonstration where the students had an opportunity to handle the related equipment. She had noticed that one of the first-year students, Aisha, didn't seem to be learning this skill as well as the others. Sumatra has started to write a reflective entry in her journal about this.

I just couldn't think why Aisha didn't seem to understand what I was asking her to do. She wasn't even able to answer the questions in the quiz I did at the end of the session. The other students seemed to pick it up straight away and I was really pleased with them and told them so. I could see by the puzzled look on Aisha's face during the demonstration that she was struggling with this more than the others. When I asked her to demonstrate connecting the giving set to the bag of fluids, she opened the packaging all wrong and even dropped the giving set on the floor. She just picked it up and started to attach it to the fluids without even commenting on what had happened. When I asked her if she thought that would be OK to do that for real, she just shrugged!

In Scenario 4.1 it seems that Sumatra has designed a learning activity without considering the different learning needs of the individual students attending the session. Although she has created a session that is relevant for the students, it will not be developing them as empowered or autonomous learners as it does not offer any opportunities for learning to be individualised.

Activity 4.1   Critical thinking

Using the examples of how to support learner autonomy and empowerment with your students introduced earlier in this chapter, think about how Sumatra could have better designed the session.

There is a model answer for this activity at the end of the chapter.

Learning is generally defined as a process of an individual acquiring new knowledge resulting in changes to their internal and external behaviours. Internally, learning might result in changes to an individual's way of thinking, their attitudes and their emotional responses. External changes from learning involve the observable differences, for example: how a student might professionally conduct themselves, communicate or undertake a practice task (Olson, 2015). Learning does not depend solely on the teacher or presentation of the knowledge. Instead, the student uses their own strengths and experience to enable learning to occur. You might have had a similar experience to Sumatra in Scenario 4.1 where a student hasn't seemed to have engaged in learning activities. Learning theories can help us to better understand how individuals absorb, process and retain knowledge.

Learning theories

How we learn is entirely individual and is influenced by cognitive, environmental and emotional factors. Our prior experiences as well as world view also affect how we learn, or acquire new knowledge. There are many different theories available in books and online resources about how we learn, although it is generally recognised that there are three main learning theories. These are behaviourist, cognitive constructivist and social constructivist learning theories, which are widely cited in educational text. In healthcare, two other theories are also used, namely connectivism and andragogy. Table 4.1 provides a summary of these key learning theories as well as some teaching and learning strategies related to each approach (Aliakbari et al., 2015; Olson, 2015). Once you have read through the table, Activity 4.2 provides you with an opportunity to consider your personal views of knowledge and learning in light of these theories. Understanding learning theories and our own particular views about learning can help us to be more effective in supporting our students to learn as well as empowering them as autonomous learners (Olson, 2015).

Learning theory	View of knowledge and learning	Associated learning theorists (major theorists are in bold)	Key principles of how learning happens	Motivations for learning	Helpful teaching and learning strategies
Behaviourism	*Knowledge and learning are behavioural responses to environmental stimuli.*	**Ivan Pavlov, B. F. Skinner,** Albert Bandura, John B. Watson, E.L. Thorndike	Learning is the acquisition of new behaviours based on environmental conditions. Humans and animals learn in the same way. Learning involves a behavioural change which is objectively observable. The teacher is *active* and learner is *passive*.	The teacher uses a stimuli to obtain a response, and rewards the learner once they have positively responded.	Compliment and praise good/ desired behaviours. Support the praise with evidence and examples wherever possible – for example, colleague or patient/ service user feedback. Utilise negative reinforcement. For example, if the student is displaying inappropriate professional behaviours, remove any opportunities for additional placement visits and activities until the desired behaviours are displayed.
Cognitive constructivism	*Knowledge and learning is a process of acquiring and storing information.*	**Jean Piaget,** William G. Perry, William Cobern, David A. Kolb, John Dewey	Mental structures (thus learning) are created from earlier structures, and not directly from environmental information. What happens *inside one's head* is more important than observable behaviours.	Motivation is largely intrinsic as it involves significant personal investment on the part of the learner. Learners become aware of the limitations in their existing knowledge and accept the need to add to or modify this existing knowledge.	Encourage the student to identify their own learning needs and how to pursue these (to *construct* learning). Encourage active participation in relevant activities. Identify the student's interests and build this into any learning experiences.

(Continued)

Table 4.1 (Continued)

Learning theory	View of knowledge and learning	Associated learning theorists (major theorists are in bold)	Key principles of how learning happens	Motivations for learning	Helpful teaching and learning strategies
			Knowledge is not passively transmitted from the environment to the learner. Instead the learner is *active* as a *maker of meaning*. Learning happens by applying previously acquired skills and knowledge to a new situation. This might involve adjusting previously acquired skills and knowledge, or accommodating new skills and knowledge, to better understand the situation.		Ask students to explain new material or experiences in their own words and assist them in assimilating this as they re-express the new ideas in their own language. Ask students to self-assess their own performance. Utilise problem-based-learning, reflection and concept mapping learning strategies. As a teacher, facilitate and guide learning as opposed to imparting lots of information.
Social constructivism	*All cognitive functions originate in, so must then be explained as, products of social interactions.* There is a variety of cognitive constructivism that places an increased emphasis on the collaborative nature of learning.	Lev Vygotsky	Learning is not just the assimilation and accommodation of new knowledge by learners, but the process by which learners are integrated into a wider *knowledge community*. Language and culture play essential roles in human intellectual development and in how humans perceive the world. These are social phenomena, thus knowledge is socially built *(co-constructed)*.	Motivation is both extrinsic and intrinsic. Learners are partially motivated by the rewards provided by the wider knowledge community and as knowledge is constructed by the individual they must have an internal drive to learn.	Facilitate group learning, encourage discussion based around a topic. With the student, identify a learning need and introduce them to the idea of networking with relevant individuals to help them learn about this. Follow up self-directed learning activities with discussions to further develop understanding, maybe presenting learning back to the wider team and giving encouraging comments.

Connectivism			
In our digital society, the connections and connectiveness within networks lead to learning. This is a variety of social constructivism and the work of Lev Vygotsky.	**Stephen Downes** **George Siemens**	The learner's level of *actual* development is the level the learner has already reached, and where they are capable of solving problems independently. The learner's level of potential development is the level the learner is capable of reaching under the guidance of teachers or working in collaboration with peers. This is where learning takes place. Learning occurs through connections within (digital) networks and by connecting to and growing personal networks. Learners learn through recognising and interpreting patterns. (Knowledge-based) decisions are based on rapidly altering foundations. New information is continually being acquired so there is a necessity to draw distinctions between important and unimportant information.	Use online resources that also offer online discussion forums. Facilitate a group debriefing at the end of a shift or after a particular incident. Utilise action learning sets, group work, and peer learning strategies. As a teacher, facilitate and guide learning with and from relevant others, as opposed to imparting lots of information.
		A learner's capacity to know more is more critical than what is currently known. A strong motivator is the diversity of the learner's networks, strength of ties and the context of their network.	Support the student in making new/maintaining relevant networking connections. An example might be connecting to other professionals in their field through workplace social media platforms. Support the student to improve their digital capabilities relevant to their developing practice. Signpost the student to evidence-based and research-informed practices.

(Continued)

Table 4.1 (Continued)

Learning theory	View of knowledge and learning	Associated learning theorists (major theorists are in bold)	Key principles of how learning happens	Motivations for learning	Helpful teaching and learning strategies
			Understanding of a particular area or field will happen more quickly if individuals are connected to networks, building evidence-based repositories. The potential to learn does not reside solely within humans and animals, but also within technologies.		Nurture the student's ability to see connections between ideas, and concepts as a core skill. Model how decisions are made within an ever-changing environment, and support the student in recognising quality data sources to help inform clinical decision-making.
Adult learning theory (andragogy)	*Adults learn differently to children and naturally tend to be more self-directed, internally motivated, and ready to learn.*	**Malcolm Knowles**	Adults are at a mature developmental stage thus having a more secure *self-concept* than children. This enables them to take a greater part in directing their learning. Adults have a breadth of experiences to draw upon while they learn. Learning should therefore add to what is already known and build upon prior knowledge. Commonly, adults are involved in practical learning. Therefore learning should focus on/make explicit the links to issues related to practice.	Adults are internally motivated because: • many adults have reached a point in which they see the value of education and are ready to learn; • many adults return to learning for specific practical reasons, such as entering a new role.	Explain or provide the reasons and rationale for what is being taught. Any instruction should be linked and applied to practice examples and task-oriented instead of promoting memorising facts or knowledge. Teachers should take into account the wide range of different backgrounds of students, levels and learning styles to facilitate students to build on/link to existing knowledge and skills wherever possible. Adult students are self-directed, so any instruction should allow them to discover new knowledge for themselves. Utilise problem-based learning and self-directed approaches.

Table 4.1 Summary of key learning theories

Activity 4.2 Reflection

Take a few moments to think about your view of knowledge and learning and how learning happens for you. Is there one of the theories outlined in Table 4.1 that you feel best fits with your views? You might wish to make a note of this for your portfolio.

There is no model answer for this activity as it relates to your own views. However, if you would like to read more about theories of knowledge and learning and how learning happens, please access the further reading listed at the end of the chapter, in particular Aliakbari et al. (2015). This article outlines some commonly used theories in nursing and midwifery education, as well as the associated benefits and disadvantages.

The theories outlined in Table 4.1 have substantial differences in their views of knowledge and learning. The most significant difference is the theorists' views of how learning happens. One view is that knowledge is transmitted from teacher to student (behaviourist) while others view knowledge as something to be created within the individual (constructivists). This difference is because of the theorists' underlying philosophical thinking about the scope and nature of knowledge. Our underlying philosophical ideas will affect how we approach teaching and learning. Did you recognise which theory your views identified in Activity 4.2 most aligned with?

Each of the learning theories, as well as others not mentioned here, will have influenced and shaped educational practices in your clinical practice setting in some way. If we think about Sumatra's session in Scenario 4.1, she delivered some content that the students committed to memory and then were expected to complete an assessment (in the form of a quiz) of their learning at the end. When the students did well (desired behaviour) Sumatra rewarded them by giving them positive feedback as she was *really pleased with them and told them so.* We can see how this would fit with a behaviourist approach.

If Sumatra chooses to next ask Aisha to assess her own performance during that practical and then identify her learning needs before undertaking another assessment with this task, she could be utilising a constructivist approach. If she facilitates a group practical with all the students where they work on the same task and are encouraged to discuss their developing learning, it could be viewed as a social constructivist approach. From this example we can see how practice supervisors and assessors use approaches from learning theories in an integrated way to complement the particular learning experience. Educators are better equipped to support students and handle a variety of learning situations, with some understanding of these approaches.

Other learning theories have also been developed for more specific purposes, for example theories about the learning style we ourselves identify with.

Learning styles

The underlying principle of all learning styles, theories and frameworks is that individuals learn but in different ways and at different levels. Different learning style theories focus on: how students process information, how students acquire information or preferences towards cognitive modalities. Although different theorists use different tools, usually a set of questions is asked, and our responses identify our preferred learning style. Being aware of different learning styles can:

- help students to understand which opportunities will best help them to learn. This can help to accelerate their learning, and make learning more effective and enjoyable.
- expand on the experiences students access. Going beyond activities linked to a student's *preferred* style will help them to become an *all-rounder*, which will maximise their learning opportunities.
- support educators in planning opportunities which contain activities to suit students across all styles, encouraging maximum engagement.

There are many learning styles theories, frameworks and models available. One commonly used learning style theory was developed by Peter Honey and Alan Mumford (2000) and uses a questionnaire to identify an individual's distinct learning styles or preferences. They suggest that individuals naturally identify with *styles* of being an activist, theorist, pragmatist or reflector. They explain the characteristics of each of these styles are:

Activists (doers)

- immerse themselves fully in new experiences;
- enjoy the here and now;
- are open minded, enthusiastic, flexible;
- act first, then consider the consequences later;
- seek to centre an activity around themselves.

Reflectors (reviewers)

- stand back and observe;
- are cautious, like to take a back seat;
- collect and analyse data about experience and events, and are slow to reach conclusions;
- use information from past, present and immediate observations to maintain a big picture perspective.

Theorists (concluders)

- think through problems in a logical manner and value rationality and objectivity;
- can assimilate disparate facts into coherent theories;
- are disciplined, aiming to fit things into a rational order;
- are keen on basic assumptions, principles, theories, models and systems thinking.

Pragmatists (planners)

- are keen to put ideas, theories and techniques into practice;
- will search out new ideas and like to experiment;
- can act quickly and confidently on ideas, getting straight to the point;
- are impatient with endless discussion.

There are many websites where you can take Honey and Mumford's (2000) learning styles test, or other similar learning styles questionnaires. You might try undertaking one of these yourself to help you identify your own learning style. Familiarising yourself with the styles will help you to recognise traits and preferences in others around you. You might even ask your student about their preferred learning style. Table 4.2 summarises the four learning styles from Honey and Mumford (2000) and how individuals identifying with each of these learn, as well as some useful related teaching activities.

Activity 4.3   Critical thinking

Take a few moments to think about your preferred learning style. Is there one of the styles from Honey and Mumford (2000) presented earlier in this chapter that you feel you most identify with? Now think about some of the students you have worked with. Can you work out what their preferred learning styles might have been from their engagement with various learning activities? How might the learning styles affect how you worked together?

You might wish to make a note of this for your portfolio.

There is no model answer for this activity as it relates to your own style and experiences.

Learning styles, as with any other style, are strengthened by individuals repeating particular learning strategies and tactics that they have then found to work for them. Certain behaviours develop that then become habitual. Individuals may gravitate towards certain roles or career choices that fit with their preferred style. Honey and Mumford (2000) suggest that because of this, it is useful for students to be challenged with a range of activities to encourage them to be *all-rounders*. In Activity 4.3 did you strongly identify with any particular learning styles and could you recognise any of these traits in the students you have worked with? It is likely that we will be regularly supporting students who have a different style to our own. We might find our own style differs at different points of our career. An awareness of different preferences to learning and providing variation in our activities is critical.

	Activists	Reflectors	Theorists	Pragmatists
Learn best from or actively look for activities where they have ...	new experiences and challenges from which to learn	permission or encouragement to watch/think/ponder on activities	ideas offered which are part of a system, model, concept, theory or evidence base	been given an obvious link between the subject matter and a *real life* problem
	short *here and now* tasks involving competitive team work and problem-solving approaches	time to think before acting, to assimilate before commenting	time to explore methodically the associations and interrelationships between ideas, events and situations	been shown techniques for doing things with obvious practical advantages
	excitement, change and variety	opportunities to carry out careful, detailed research	opportunity to question and probe the basic methodology, assumptions or logic	the chance to try out and practise techniques with coaching or feedback from a credible expert
	high-visibility tasks such as chairing meetings, leading discussions and presentations	time to review their learning	opportunity to be intellectually stretched, e.g; by being asked to analyse and evaluate, then generalise	a model they can emulate, or examples/anecdotes
	situations in which new ideas can be developed without constraints of policy and structure	time to produce carefully considered analyses and reports	a part in structured situations with a clear purpose	been given techniques currently applicable to their own work
	opportunities for just *having a go*	help to exchange views with other people without danger, by prior agreement, within a structured learning experience	visions presented, see interesting ideas and concepts, whether or not they are immediately relevant	immediate opportunities to implement what they have learnt
		opportunity to reach a decision without pressure and tight deadlines		time to concentrate on practical issues, such as drawing up action plans or giving tips to others
Learn least from or may avoid activities where they have ...	a passive role (for example, lectures, instructions, reading)	felt *forced* into the limelight	no apparent context or purpose	been presented with learning that is not related to an immediate need they recognise
	a role as observers	felt they must act without time for planning	to participate in situations emphasising emotions and feelings	organisers of the learning who they think are distant from reality
	to assimilate, analyse and interpret lots of *messy* data	been asked for an instant reaction, or *off the cuff* thoughts	to be involved in unstructured activities where ambiguity and uncertainty are high	no clear guidelines
	to work in a solitary way (for example, reading and writing alone)	been given insufficient data on which to base a conclusion	been asked to act or decide without a basis in policy, principle or concept	

statements that are *theoretical* – providing an explanation of cause considerable repetition (for example, practising the same skill) precise instructions with little room for manoeuvre a requirement to be thorough, and tie up loose ends	had to make short cuts or do a superficial job, in the interests of expediency	been presented with a hotchpotch of alternative or contradictory techniques or methods without exploring any in depth doubt that the subject matter is methodologically sound a feeling of being out of tune with other participants, for example when they are with lots of activists	a feeling that people are going round in circles rather than getting to the point political, organisational, managerial or personal obstacles to implementation no apparent reward from the learning activity (for example, higher grades)
Examples of useful teaching activities include... hands on, practical experiences, demonstrations simulation, role play brainstorming, mapping group discussions, debate puzzles, games, competitions	time out to process new information, skills etc. paired or group discussions debriefing after events self-analysis, self-assessment and self-evaluation multiple observation opportunities for practice skills feedback from others including peers, supervisors and patients/service users regular meetings in a coaching, mentoring, clinical supervisor relationship	working through evidence base, research, pathways, guidelines models, statistics quotes, stories, talking heads, patient feedback background information, case notes, resource files opportunity to apply theories	opportunities to put learning into practice in the real world opportunity to try out new ideas, theories and techniques to see if they work time to think about how to apply learning in reality case studies, with real life examples problem solving paired or group discussion regular meetings with practice supervisor

Table 4.2 Summary of learning styles

Activity 4.4   Critical thinking

Look at Scenario 4.1; it seems that Aisha's preferred learning style has not been accounted for in Sumatra's session. From your understanding of Honey and Mumford's (2000) learning styles presented earlier in this chapter:

1.   What might be Sumatra's preferred learning style?
2.   What might be Aisha's preferred learning style? What types of activities would best suit this style?

There is a model answer at the end of this chapter.

Although learning styles are widely used within healthcare education, their effectiveness has been criticised by some authors. Over the years there have been claims that: learning style measures are weak in reliability and validity, can be confusing to use and are based upon little evidence (Willingham et al., 2015). However, many studies focusing on nursing and midwifery students have shown the importance of teachers adapting their approaches to students' preferences. When teaching strategies are congruent to learning style preferences, students are more motivated to learn, feel responsibility for their own learning, achieved high grades and have higher satisfaction with their courses (Hallin, 2014). Understanding learning styles and related activities suited to different styles can therefore be incredibly helpful. When we are planning learning activities, the key is to ensure that we cover a range of activities that will help to engage and challenge our students.

Learning with peers

Students working together in a learning environment will be involved in similar experiences and will engage intellectually, emotionally and socially in *constructive conversation*. Learning occurs by talking and questioning each other's views to reach agreements or divides (Boud et al., 2014). This is something that occurs naturally. You might have noticed that if a student has a question, they will often intuitively ask another student. Students often feel safer going to a peer than a supervisor or assessor whose experience or position might make them intimidating. A peer is closer to the student's own position and level of experience, so is more likely to have had similar questions and think in a similar way.

Peer learning is an educational approach available to practice supervisors, assessors and educators. It describes how students learn *with*, *from* and *about* each other, and is very current in the shift from teacher-focused to student-focused education. We can use this naturally occurring phenomenon by building in opportunities for peer learning wherever possible. Peer learning is usually associated with **communities of practice** and the work of the social constructivist educational theorists. Instead of viewing learning as an individual process and as a result of teaching, peer learning assumes students construct their own meaning and understanding of what they need to learn. This is an essential component for students to become empowered in their learning and be autonomous learners. This approach is supported by the rise in the use of information technologies providing students with increased opportunities to learn and access networks. Activity 4.5 encourages you to think of peer learning opportunities in your clinical practice area.

Activity 4.5   Reflection

Can you think of a time when students in your clinical practice area learnt together, or when you learnt with your peers? If so, did you notice any benefits from peer learning?

You might want to make a note of this in your portfolio.

There is a model answer at the end of this chapter.

Peer learning is about much more than gaining content knowledge. It is a student-centred approach that can provide a richer student experience that effectively prepares the student for their professional roles as well as the diversity of workplace. Peer learning has gained significant momentum over recent years in health professional education and has a strong evidence base supporting its efficacy and benefits. Studies have shown that students find it acceptable, enjoyable and helpful to learning. In addition, peer learning can develop a student's skills in teaching and supervision, as well as in giving feedback (Boud et al., 2014). Peer learning has also been linked to **self-efficacy** or the individual's belief in their ability to succeed; the creation of a feeling of responsibility towards one's own learning and learner empowerment (Palsson et al., 2017). You might have noted some of these benefits in Activity 4.5.

In Scenario 4.1, Sumatra could use peer learning to encourage the students to support each other with development of the new skill in her session. It is likely that some of the students in her group will have either seen or undertaken this skill previously, or have some knowledge to share relating to this. As supervisors and assessors, we can build in opportunities for our students to work together, encouraging peer learning wherever possible. As with most educational approaches, it works best when planned carefully and used appropriately. Peer learning should supplement time spent with a practice supervisor or assessor and never be used to replace that level of support.

Interprofessional learning

Interprofessional education (IPE) is widely understood and defined as *two or more professions learning with, from and about each other to improve collaboration and quality of care* (Atkins, 2002). It remains a key component of healthcare policy, supported by governments, healthcare regulators and academic institutions. IPE is recognised as having the benefits for peer learning introduced earlier in this chapter, as well as being a means to improve collaborative and interprofessional practice in the workplace. It adds an additional dimension to peer learning, by adding another or other professional lens/lenses. As well as learning about one's own professional context, students learn from each about other professional context, to support a more joined up and holistic approach to care. The World Health Organisation (WHO) (2013) makes clear the link with IPE and collaborative practice in healthcare. In their report *Interprofessional collaborative practice in primary health care: nursing and midwifery perspectives* (WHO, 2013), they use six case studies in order to identify the enabling mechanisms and barriers to IPE. Activity 4.6 provides a summary of barriers to IPE and is useful for us to think about our own learning environments.

Activity 4.6   Evidence-based practice

Read this section adapted from *Interprofessional collaborative practice in primary health care: nursing and midwifery perspectives* (WHO, 2013). Think about if any of these barriers are relevant in your clinical practice area.

Section 6.2 Summary of barriers in case studies

Professional cultures and stereotypes

In the process of establishing unique professional identities, healthcare professionals often overlook the value of teamwork and collaboration. Numerous studies have found evidence of professional cultures and stereotypes being adopted by health professionals. One of the most prevalent stereotypes among physicians is that they see themselves as *leaders* and *decision-makers* whereas other healthcare professionals are considered to be *team players*. Recognising that these stereotypes and attitudes become more entrenched with time, a number of scholars have emphasised the importance of addressing students' beliefs and assumptions early in their professional training. The Brazilian and Canadian case studies demonstrate initiatives introducing mandatory IPE programmes early in health professional curricula; other case study settings do not have this IPE requirement.

Inconsistent use and different understandings of language

A wide range of terminology is used interchangeably to describe Collaborative Practice (CP); health professionals also have different understandings of what it means to *collaborate*. All the case studies showed that inconsistent use of language concerning CP and related concepts resulted in inconsistency in reporting CP-related issues, which made data gathering and analysis more challenging.

Accreditation and curricula

Accreditation bodies for health professions determine what is included and what excluded from their curricula. Successful implementation of CP requires the inclusion of IPE in accreditation and registration requirements. While accreditation was not a focus in the case studies, participants in India commented on accreditation by government or educational institutions, and defined accreditation as the continuing assessment of staff/volunteers by methods including feedback, testing and review processes.

Shared vision

A shared vision was identified as a key enabler in the literature, helping to unify a team, and facilitating the achievement of its common goals. While all the programmes studied here define their goals, they do not label these as a shared vision. Only programme-specific goals were described, such as providing comprehensive HIV care, helping to fill existing gaps in healthcare systems, and promoting relationships between academics, the community and health services in PHC, as well as goals on IPE for CP.

There is no model answer to this activity as it relates to your practice setting.

You might have identified particular barriers to IPE in your own practice setting in Activity 4.6, but what makes for a successful IPE learning environment?

Being aware of our own professional cultures and stereotypes; using consistent language; understanding how IPE fits with the curricula and creating a shared vision are fundamental in the success of IPE. The literature also suggests that students get the greatest benefits from IPE when they direct the learning experiences and opportunities are student-focused. The learning experience should be realistic and patient/client-centred as this provides the perfect learning environment for IPE (McDonough, 2016). However, IPE requires good facilitation. If we are working with students from two or more professional backgrounds examples of learning experiences we could plan include: patient/client-centred case conferences ward rounds; hand overs; debriefing events after care episodes or specific events; group reflection or action learning sets. In our roles as practice supervisors and assessors, we are ideally placed to ensure that IPE learning is developed and consolidated.

There are many ways in which we can develop our students to be empowered and autonomous learners. Considering their individual learning preferences and styles as well as creating peer and interprofessional learning opportunities are all key. Another consideration we need to be mindful of is the link between the student's generation and their potential learning preference.

Effects of 'generation' on learning

Different generations can be viewed as having unique cultures and characteristics, which in turn can shape their beliefs and expectations. This includes generational differences in approaches to learning. A report commissioned by Health Education England (HEE) called *Mind the gap: exploring the needs of early career nurses and midwives in the workplace* (Jones et al., 2015) outlines the different characteristics of each generation and is summarised in Table 4.3 (NHS Employers, 2017).

Generation	'Baby boomers' born 1946–1954	'Generation X' born 1965–1980	'Generation Y' born 1981–1994	'Generation Z' born 1995–2010
Characteristics	Motivated and hardworking; define self-worth by their work and accomplishments	Practical self-starters, but work–life balance is important to them	Ambitious, with high career expectations; need mentorship and reassurance	Highly innovative, but will expect to be informed. Personal freedom is essential
Percentage of the NHS workforce	25%	44%	25%	6%
Attitude towards technology	Early Information Technology (IT) adopters	Digital immigrants	Digital natives	'Technoholics' – dependent on IT and little knowledge of alternatives

Communication preferences	Face to face, but telephone or email if necessary	Text messaging or email	Online and mobile (texting)	Facetime, Snapchat
Attitude towards career	Careers are defined and shaped by their employers	Loyal to their profession but not necessarily their employers	Working *with* organisations but not necessarily *for*	Career multitaskers, can switch easily between roles, more likely to have multiple careers

Table 4.3   Overview of characteristics of generations

Generation Z is now entering undergraduate nursing and midwifery programmes and starting to become registrants. These will bring some different life characteristics from those of their practice supervisors and assessors who they are working with. These students will have a tendency to prefer experiential learning and teaching methods for example *how to* videos of clinical skills, and working with passionate educators. Multiple resources must be quickly available to them for them to be able to search and find answers. Seeing students using the internet and messaging constantly can be frustrating, but can be used as a useful learning resource. However, using the internet and messaging for personal use while in the workplace environment can create patient safety risks and should be discouraged. The NMC Code (2015) is useful to refer to if this becomes an issue with your student. The average Generation Z student will have an attention span of 8 seconds, which is much shorter than previous generations. They are likely to use the first information they get as they are looking for instant *answers* so guidance on good and reliable evidence is required.

Generation Z students like learning in groups and in social settings, as well as working independently at their own pace with resources tailored to their needs. They will like teaching strategies using technology as well as practical application, for example, problem-based learning, simulation and role play. As well as the differences in learning styles, the impact of these generational characteristics might be at play for Sumatra and her group of students in the scenario. The key is offering choice wherever possible.

The potential impact of the generational differences is nicely summarised in the extract from the summary of *Mind the Gap: Exploring the Needs of Early Career Nurses and Midwives in the Workplace* (Jones et al., 2015, p3), which helps us to think about the potential impact of the generational differences.

Through this work we have learnt that there are generational concepts that require consideration if we are to appropriately support individuals as they begin their professional careers. For the first time in history four different generations will be working together in the same employment environment. There are generational differences in values, expectations, perceptions and motivations in the current workforce and these are highly relevant in terms of staff education and engagement. Understanding differing motivational needs across these generations offers employers and education providers a real opportunity to better align support to meet individual needs and to improve recruitment and retention.

Chapter summary

This chapter has introduced you to the key concepts of student empowerment and autonomy. It has provided an overview of the literature around learning theories and style. By completing the activities you have considered how your preferred learning style might impact upon how you and your students learn. Through the chapter scenario, we noted how understanding learning styles and theories can equip practice supervisors and assessors to individualise learning. Given the increased focus on interprofessional working in healthcare, we considered the benefits of peer and interprofessional learning as well as the links between student empowerment and collaborative practice. The chapter concluded by introducing another aspect that could influence student learning, namely the impact of *generation*.

Activity answers

Activity 4.1: Critical thinking (p60)

Using the examples of how to support learner autonomy and empowerment with your students introduced earlier in this chapter, Sumatra could:

- Provide an opportunity for students to request the content of any sessions, arising from their needs. When the content is necessary or mandatory for the clinical area, design the session with opportunities for student initiated question asking.
- Ask the students in the session to begin by talking about what they already know and the skills they have already gained relating to intravenous infusions. Ensure the students are aware that what is disclosed in the session is confidential, in case previous negative experiences are discussed. Encourage them to highlight areas they need to focus on during this learning opportunity.
- Provide opportunity in the session for students to work with other students, mixing levels of experience wherever possible.
- Plan activities that help the student to have impact, for example, talking through their demonstration of the skill to Sumatra and other students.
- Introduce any jargon and acronyms that are related to this skill, encourage students to note any of these which are unfamiliar.
- Positively encourage participation, creating an atmosphere of mutual respect.
- Provide time for students to discuss the skill, introducing any relevant evidence, policy, guidelines supporting it.

Activity 4.4: Critical thinking (p70)

1. Sumatra might be an activist as the session she has designed has lots of activities designed for that preferred style.

2. We do not have enough detail to know exactly which learning style Aisha most identifies with. Aisha might require more time to reflect on the demonstration of the skill or to be able to see additional demonstrations (reflector). She might need to understand the underlying theory behind the skill, apply some of her related knowledge including fluid management and aseptic techniques, before being able to undertake the skill herself (theorist). Sumatra could use her understanding of learning styles to offer additional learning activities for Aisha. When she plans for future teaching sessions she should ensure that she covers a range of activities to engage students with different styles.

Activity 4.5: Reflection (p71)

There is no specific answer to this activity because these are your own personal reflections. However, you might have noted that peer learning is most effective when students are given an opportunity to get together to learn in small, collaborative groups. This might have been built into shift patterns or informally arranged. You can support peer learning by building into your students' work arrangements opportunities for them to meet with other students. You might have also noted that for peer learning to be effective, the group must have mutual respect, confidence and trust for one another. Each member must feel able to participate and have their voice heard. You can support peer learning by helping the setup of groups with introductions and ground rules.

You might have noted some of the following benefits:

- self-directed learning skills (associated with student autonomy and empowerment);
- motivated students;
- critical thinking and problem-solving skills;
- interpersonal and team working skills;
- critical reflection skills;
- friendships and the social aspects of learning, tips and *survival skills* to help each other learn to nurse;
- peer teaching and assessment, especially found in clinical skill acquisition.

Further reading

Aliakbari, F, Parvin, N, Heidari, M and Haghani, F (2015) Learning theories application in nursing education. *Journal of Education and Health Promotion*, 4.

This article is a systematic review of the relevant literature, which combines learning theories research and nurse education. It outlines some commonly used theories as well as the associated benefits and disadvantages.

Davis, E and Richardson, S (2017) How peer facilitation can help nursing students develop their skills. *British Journal of Nursing*, 26(21): 1187–91.

This article reports on the implementation of a peer facilitation scheme for pre-registration nurses. It offers an insight into how to implement this sort of scheme, as well as benefits that were noted.

Chapter 5 — Supervisors, assessors and educators

Standards Framework for Nursing and Midwifery Education. Part 1 of Realising Professionalism: Standards for Education and Training (NMC, 2018d)

This chapter will address the standards in heading **4: Educators and assessors**.

4.1 Theory and practice learning and assessment are facilitated effectively and objectively by an appropriately qualified and experienced professional with necessary expertise for their educational and assessor roles.

The Code: professional standards of practice and behaviour for nurses and midwives (NMC, 2015)

This chapter most closely aligns with the following professional standards.

Practise effectively

6.1 make sure that any information or advice given is evidence-based, including information relating to using any healthcare products or services.

6.2 maintain the knowledge and skills you need for safe and effective practice.

7.1 use terms that people in your care, colleagues and the public can understand.

8.1 respect the skills, expertise and contributions of your colleagues, referring matters to them when appropriate.

8.2 maintain effective communication with colleagues.

8.4 work with colleagues to evaluate the quality of your work and that of the team.

9.1 provide honest, accurate and constructive feedback to colleagues.

9.2 gather and reflect on feedback from a variety of sources, using it to improve your practice and performance.

9.4 support students' and colleagues' learning to help them develop their professional competence and confidence.

10.1 complete all records at the time or as soon as possible after an event, recording if the notes are written sometime after the event.

11.1   only delegate tasks and duties that are within the other person's scope of competence, making sure that they fully understand your instructions.

11.2   make sure that everyone you delegate tasks to is adequately supervised and supported so they can provide safe and compassionate care.

11.3   confirm that the outcome of any task you have delegated to someone else meets the required standard.

13.5   complete the necessary training before carrying out a new role.

Promote professionalism and trust

20.3   be aware at all times of how your behaviour can affect and influence the behaviour of other people.

20.8   act as a role model of professional behaviour for students and newly qualified nurses and midwives to aspire to.

25.2   support any staff you may be responsible for to follow the Code at all times. They must have the knowledge, skills and competence for safe practice; and understand how to raise any concerns linked to any circumstances where the Code has, or could be, broken.

Chapter aims

After reading this chapter, you will be able to:

- understand the skills and attributes required to be a practice supervisor and assessor;
- recognise the purpose, benefits and principles of collaboratively supporting student learning in practice;
- articulate the benefits of using learning objectives and identifying student needs for maximising learning opportunities;
- develop an understanding of common teaching methods helpful for your role.

Introduction

In this chapter we meet Mike who is a newly qualified registrant, looking forward to becoming involved in supporting students in his practice area. He is starting to plan to undertake the practice supervisor preparation required by his organisation. We are introduced to skills and attributes required for this role, and consider the overlaps with other skills and attributes Mike may already possess. We consider the benefits of working collaboratively to support students with their learning, as well as some of the principles involved in making this successful. Developing and using learning objectives and identifying students' needs are covered, as well as considering how these inform learning opportunities that are available. The chapter outlines common teaching methods used in clinical areas to support the student when applying theoretical knowledge to practice. The advantages and disadvantages associated with these are outlined, as well as the role of reflection for the practice supervisor/assessor.

Scenario 5.1

Mike is coming towards the end of his preceptorship period as a newly qualified nurse. He thoroughly enjoyed his time as a student nurse and although he found the initial transition to becoming a registered nurse difficult, he loves being a nurse and enjoys the ward where he's currently working. He has noticed that lots of the students on his ward often request to work with him, and ask him for advice or information. Last week a third-year student Anil started, who asked Mike if he would be his practice supervisor. He said to Mike that he found him to be *really approachable* and loved his enthusiasm for nursing. Mike was pleased to be asked, but knew that he had to decline. Unfortunately, he has not yet worked through the training package for practice supervisors that he needs to complete in preparation for the role, in his particular organisation.

Mike really enjoys working with students and has recently identified with his preceptor that he would like to do more of this. He thinks back to nurses that supervised and assessed him when he was a student and compares himself to how they were. He is anticipating there will be a lot to learn and he might not be able to fulfil the role requirements. One of his colleagues had said to him that he needed *years of experience* before he should be supervising students. Although he knows from the NMC education standards this is not true, it has made him a little apprehensive. However, he plans to start working through the learning package, and has spoken with the educational lead in his organisation about this.

Preparation for becoming a practice supervisor and practice assessor

In Scenario 5.1, Mike is planning to undertake his practice supervisor training but has been told by a colleague he needs more experience. He clearly is able to fulfil these roles, once he has undertaken suitable preparation, as supported by his local work area and AEI. It is a myth that the number of years a health professional has been in their role equates to how good they will be at supporting practice learning. Many students enjoy working with more experienced students or newly qualified registrants. They probably feel that as they have recently been in their position, they are better placed to understand their needs and how to support them.

The NMC (2018b) states that the practice supervisor can be *any registered health and social care professional* who is supporting and supervising learning in practice in line with their competence. In addition, practice assessors are NMC-registered nurses or midwives who have been suitably prepared and receive on-going support to perform their role. More about these roles is detailed in Chapter 1. However, the NMC do not prescribe an NMC-approved preparation programme for either of these roles as they have done in the past. The preparation requirements for both of these roles are outlined in Table 5.1.

	Preparation for practice supervisor role	Preparation for practice assessor role
Approved education institutions, together with practice learning partners must ensure that practice supervisors/assessors:	receive ongoing support to prepare, reflect and develop for effective supervision and contribution to student learning and assessment, and	undertake preparation or evidence prior learning and experience that enables them to demonstrate achievement of the following minimum outcomes:
	have understanding of the proficiencies and programme outcomes they are supporting students to achieve	interpersonal communication skills, relevant to student learning and assessment
		conducting objective, evidence based assessments of students
		providing constructive feedback to facilitate professional development in others, and
		knowledge of the assessment process and their role within it

Table 5.1 Preparation requirements for practice supervisor and practice assessor roles (NMC, 2018b)

The NMC (2018b) requirements for practice supervisor and practice assessor roles as outlined in Table 5.1 are a helpful starting point for us to consider our suitability for these roles. Further exploring the skills and attributes required for these roles can help us recognise transferable skills we already have as well as any development needs.

Skills and attributes required for the roles

There are a range of factors that influence student learning in practice. These include the quality of the supervisor–student relationship and the supervisor and/or assessor's skills and attributes. Supervisors and assessors need to develop and refine a set of skills and personal attributes to enable them to effectively undertake the role. Table 5.2 summarises the key skills and attributes required when supporting student nurses and midwives in the practice area (Eller et al., 2014; Robinson et al., 2012; Huybrecht et al., 2011; Chandan and Watts, 2012). These represent key skills and attributes identified by both students and those in roles supporting practice learning.

Skills	Attributes
Facilitative of learning, providing guidance	Positive attitude
Experienced and clinically competent	Passionate and inspirational
Able to give and receive feedback	Approachable, patient and enthusiastic
A positive role model	Mutually respectful and trusting
Good time management skills, and creates space and availability	Kind, caring, compassionate
A good communicator	Committed to supporting practice education
Reflective of own practice	Confidence in their professional identity

Table 5.2 Key skills and attributes required to support student nurses and midwives in the practice area

You will notice that many of these skills and attributes presented in Table 5.2 are required for your professional role, and that you have some of these already. You might need to further develop these and begin to apply them in a different context; moving from patient application to student or learner. In Scenario 5.1, we can expect that Mike already has some of these skills and attributes, and students regularly ask to work with him. For example, Anil told Mike he was *really approachable and loved his enthusiasm for nursing*. As students have previously asked to work with Mike, we can see the importance students place on these sorts of attributes. A large-scale study of key components of an effective **mentoring** relationship (Eller et al., 2014) found that *infectious enthusiasm and passion for the work* was one of the most important factors that students cited. It is likely that Mike's local learning package will reflect these attributes and range of skills. It is important to include these attributes in preparation for the role, as well as skill development. Activity 5.1 will help you identify your own skills and attributes as well as identifying any development needs.

Activity 5.1   Reflection

Consider the list of skills and attributes in Table 5.2 and if there are any others you feel are important in order to successfully support a range of students in your practice area. Next reflect on this list and decide whether you already have these skills and attributes or whether you need to develop them further.

Consider also how you acquired these skills and attributes as this might help you develop any new ones. It will be useful to make a note of these.

There is no correct answer to this activity, as it depends on your own experience and skills. However, at the end of this chapter there are suggestions as to how you might get feedback on your skills and attributes from others, if you are not sure.

Students learn and develop their own skills, behaviours and attributes through observing their supervisors' behaviours including communicating with patients, carers and other health professions; problem solving; prioritising and decision-making strategies. Each practice learning encounter instils values and qualities in students that will shape how they professionally develop and go on to work with students themselves. Supervisors and assessors act as gatekeepers to the nursing and midwifery professions and with this responsibility is a duty to develop a future workforce that is fit for practice and purpose. This means we have a responsibility for providing students with a quality learning environment and to ensure that patient safety and quality standards are met. The Mid Staffordshire NHS Foundation Trust public inquiry report (Francis, 2013) highlighted the significance of staff values and behaviours when maintaining the standard of patient care. The impact that your role can have on developing the future workforce and maintaining the highest standards of care cannot be underestimated.

A collaborative approach to student learning

For many years, students have been encouraged to work with the wider multidisciplinary team to enhance their learning experience and have a greater understanding of the workforce. The NMC (2018a) states that students must *have opportunities to learn from a range of relevant people in practice learning environments, including service users, registered and nonregistered individuals, and other students as appropriate.* A collaborative approach to student support in the practice area describes a team-based approach to support. Many clinical areas have used a *team mentoring* approach to overcome issues associated with shortages of registrants prepared to support students in practice. However, the responsibilities for support, supervision and assessment have, until recently, been with the named *mentor* (NMC, 2008). The *Standards for Student Supervision and Assessment* (NMC, 2018b) has radically updated this approach. It has set out new guidance based on findings of other relevant reports and to best fit with today's climate and context. The RCN (2017b) noted that there had been specific problems with the mentor role, which included the difficulties experienced by students and mentors when registrants do not wish to be mentors. Examples include the *mentor qualification* being linked with promotion opportunities for many registrants. In addition, placement opportunities were limited based on the numbers of mentors clinical areas had. The RCN (2017b) suggested that a team or collaborative approach to supporting learning in practice can develop communities of practice that don't just rely on individual relationships.

A community of practice is a model of situational learning, a term developed by Lave and Wenger (1991). It is based on collaboration among peers, where individuals work to a common purpose, defined by knowledge rather than task. Communities of practice can develop naturally because individuals share a common interest, or they can be created with the goal of gaining knowledge related to a specific field. Through the process of sharing information and experiences, the individuals within the *community* learn from each other, providing an opportunity to develop personally and professionally. Many clinical areas and teams work and function as communities of practice. It therefore makes sense for student practice supervision to be undertaken by the broader team, and not just the responsibility of a named individual. The NMC (2018c, p97) states:

> *Practice supervision enables students to learn and safely achieve proficiency and autonomy in their professional role. All NMC registered nurses and midwives are capable of supervising students, serving as role models for safe and effective practice. Students may be supervised by other registered health and social care professionals.*

Potential challenges associated with a collaborative approach to student learning include: students missing out on learning opportunities; feeling unsupported if they are not sure who has responsibility for their supervision on a particular shift; difficulties with adjusting to working with and forming supportive relationships with different staff. To prevent these issues arising, supervisors need to allocate adequate time to discuss with the team students' progress at the end of shifts (Caldwell et al., 2008).

Even though there are some possible challenges of this approach, the benefits of working collaboratively to support student learning greatly outweigh these. Benefits of this approach include: ensuring that those who enjoy supervising students have an opportunity to do it; students learn from a diverse range of registrants; supervision is timely; students gain networking skills and better understanding of team roles. When others are able to contribute to the student's assessment decisions, the risk of bias is reduced. If they only ever work with one person students might feel that they have had an unfair assessment decision due to difficulties with an individual relationship.

The move by the NMC away from individual mentors to a more collaborative approach to supporting students in practice is supported by evidence. A review of the literature relating to best-practice in clinical midwifery student supervision models concluded that adopting a collaborative approach is beneficial to the clinical area and student experience (McKellar and Graham, 2017). It provides a democratic way of working and encourages shared leadership, allowing for learning to occur from all those involved. Although there have been few studies to show the impact of this approach on nursing and midwifery students to date, it is an approach widely used in other health professions. This approach signals that supporting students is *everyone's business*, echoed in the NMC Code (2015), which states registrants *Share your skills, knowledge and experience for the benefit of people receiving care and your colleagues.* Activity 5.2 will help you to begin to identify colleagues in your area who support students.

Activity 5.2   Reflection

Think about the area where you work and how many/what profession of colleagues you work with. Make a list and identify if they are registrants; their disciplines; whether they are non-registered practitioners or maybe they are a new type of healthcare worker.

Now think more closely about your colleagues and consider their role and responsibilities with regards to supporting students. Who could support student learning in your practice area, and in what capacity? Consider these roles individually and identify both the unique and shared features.

There is no correct answer to this activity, as it depends on your own experience and skills. However, at the end of this chapter there are suggestions as to some of the roles you might have identified.

Principles involved in student support

From undertaking Activity 5.2 you will have identified colleagues with whom you will be working collaboratively with to support student learning in your practice area. However, it is vital that one individual takes a lead role in organising the learning experience. This will be a colleague who has been prepared for the practice supervision/assessor role and might have prior mentoring experience. Studies have shown that when no one person takes a lead role, this results in a poorer learning experience for the student (McKellar and Graham, 2017). If in your practice area students will be working with a range of supervisors, they should be allocated a *lead* practice supervisor who co-ordinates the placement experience. Who undertakes this role will vary depending upon where you work, but this individual might be responsible for all the students in your placement. They will be the students' 'go to' person, should they have any queries or concerns relating to the placement. Daily supervision of students can be delegated within and across the team, and students will work under the direct/indirect supervision of a practice supervisor who is *suitably prepared* (NMC, 2018b). All staff in the work area will contribute to students' learning experiences in some remit, and provide feedback to the supervisor/supervisory team. This feedback is also critical for the practice assessor who is prepared to take responsibility for student assessment.

For this to work successfully, all staff members involved in student practice learning should understand their role in the education process. Effective communication and information sharing are central to the success of this.

The *lead* will need to consider how the placement is organised on a day-to-day basis and communicate this with the student who needs to be aware from the start who will be involved. You might find your practice setting has an area to make the teams *visible* with photos and names displayed. In Scenario 5.1, when Mike completes his preparation to become a practice supervisor, as specified by his organisation's arrangements, he is able to be part of the team supporting students in his workplace. As a member of this team, transparency and communication of the student objectives is essential. Mike will make sure that he familiarises himself with the programme of learning the student is on, as well as where they currently are in this programme. Objectives will then be planned relating to student contact with practice supervisors and assessors. Practice supervisors might adopt a coaching approach to working with the student. This involves planning in advance the types of experiences the student needs and how you can facilitate that. When Mike is working with his student, he will check with the student at the start of each shift what their objectives are for that shift. Mike can then ensure that his student has the learning opportunities to work towards these objectives, and consider who else might need to be involved. He also needs to plan how evidence of achievement will be obtained, ready for the student to share with their assessor at a later date. A method of communication should be established between the team and be accessible by all, including the student. In Mike's practice setting, the team use notes pages within the student's learning log to plan learning activities and provide feedback on progression. Being part of a larger support network for students has the additional benefit of supporting newly developing practice supervisors. Activity 5.3 will help you further consider factors involved in working collaboratively with others to support students' learning.

Activity 5.3   Evidence-based practice and research

Look through these considerations involved in having a collaborative approach to student support (adapted from Caldwell et al., 2008). Consider who has the responsibilities for the factors or issues to be considered in your workplace. Do you recognise your own responsibilities from this table? Does this highlight any additional actions that may be required for this approach to work in your practice area?

Considerations involved in having a collaborative approach to student support	Person/s responsible	Potential actions
Who will the team include? Do those individuals identified understand what's involved?	The person responsible for co-ordinating student support. This could be a clinical manager or education lead for example.	Identify the team; ensure all members understand what is involved and their role in supporting the student. Facilitate any training as necessary.
Students require clear information about the approach to student support.	Those supporting induction activities. Practice supervisors will explain this at initial student meetings.	Provide written information for students to access about this approach before and during the placement.
Students are allocated to work with suitably prepared practice supervisor/s and a practice assessor, and others.	Person responsible for co-ordinating student support.	Practice assessors will identify and facilitate other learning opportunities related to the student's learning needs.
Students need to be clear who can support their learning each shift.	Allocated practice supervisor/s are responsible for delegating student supervision and teaching.	The student's rota should be planned to work with identified practice supervisors each day.
A practice assessor is responsible for assessment of the student, with contributions from the team.	An identified practice assessor identifies and facilitates opportunities to discuss the student's progress and competence. They will obtain feedback and evidence from the team members.	Time should be allocated for discussion to inform and enable robust assessment of students. A clear communication strategy should be in place. For example a written system of communication can be used and accessed by all the team (and the student) if kept with the student's documentation.
The possibility of grievances being raised by students	An identified team member, the practice supervisor or practice assessor deals with the grievance.	Deal with any issues in accordance with NHS and/or organisational policy.

There is no correct answer to this activity, as it depends on your own experience and skills. However, at the end of this chapter there are suggestions for next steps if you have identified factors or issues where no-one in your workplace currently takes responsibility.

Identifying your role in supporting students as well as the role of others around you is helpful for you to understand the rich learning context of your particular work area. Matching this to the student's own learning needs and objectives will help you to organise the student's placements as well as to plan relevant learning activities.

Learning objectives, needs and opportunities

The roadmap for building the knowledge, skills and behaviours required for registration should be transparent so that students and all those involved with supporting their learning can understand the start and end point, as well as the steps in between. Learning objectives offer a way of breaking down learning into sizeable steps, as well as a common language to describe these.

Learning objectives are commonly used within educational courses, and students are generally familiar with them. They are used throughout university-based courses, as well as within continuing professional development courses. They are statements of the expected goal of the learning activity, or a description of the knowledge, skill or behaviour that will be acquired by the student as a result of the activity. Sometimes they are referred to as learning outcomes or learning goals. For some, the intent and value of learning objectives are not fully recognised, and they can be treated as being at odds with spontaneous learning opportunities. However, research shows that learning objectives work to improve student outcomes when teachers and students engage with them and use them as a basis for planning activities, feedback conversations, and assessments (Austin, 2018).

During conversations and meetings with your student, you can support the development of their learning objectives by ensuring that:

- a realistic number of learning objectives are set (these can always be added to during the placement if achieved);
- learning objectives take into account the level and experience of the student – they should be challenging yet achievable;
- a plan is developed of how they will be achieved, identifying potential learning opportunities, as well as how learning will be recorded.

Writing learning objectives as SMART objectives is helpful. A SMART objective is Specific, Measurable, Achievable, Realistic and Time-phased. The Department for Health and Human Services (2009) provides the following guidance for writing SMART objectives:

1. Specific:
   - Objectives should provide the *who* and *what* of learning activities.
   - Use only one action verb since objectives with more than one verb imply that more than one activity or behaviour is being measured.

- Avoid verbs that may have vague meanings to describe intended outcomes (e.g. *understand* or *know*) since it may prove difficult to measure them. Instead, use verbs that document action (e.g. *At the end of the visit, the students will list three functions of the …*).
- Remember, the greater the specificity, the greater the measurability.

2. Measurable:

   - The focus is on *how much* learning is expected.
   - Objectives should quantify the amount of learning expected.
   - It is impossible to determine whether objectives have been met unless they can be measured.
   - The objective provides a reference point from which a change can clearly be measured.

3. Achievable:

   - Objectives should be attainable within a given time frame and with available resources.

4. Realistic:

   - Objectives are most useful when they accurately address the scope of learning and steps that can be implemented within a specific time frame.
   - Objectives that do not directly relate to the overall course outcomes will not help towards achieving these outcomes.

5. Time-phased:

   - Objectives should provide a time frame indicating when the objective will be measured or a time by which the objective will be met.
   - Including a time frame in the objectives helps in planning and evaluating the learning experience.

Activity 5.4   Critical thinking

The characters we met in Scenario 5.1 then go on to work together as part of a wider care team during a shift. Anil discusses at the start of the shift a learning objective he has previously developed with his practice supervisor. He explains to Mike that he would like to work on this objective today. The objective is: *I will plan and deliver care on my own to a group of patients.*

1. Is this a SMART objective?
2. Write a new objective for Anil based on his ideas and what you have learnt about SMART objectives.

There is a model answer to this activity at the end of the chapter.

Working with a SMART learning outcome makes it easier for students to communicate what they are aiming to achieve as well as clearly articulating intentions to practice supervisors and assessors. Ensuring our students' objectives are SMART from the start is an important step as this will help us provide support and feedback on learning and progress.

The term *learning needs* describes the gap between a student's current knowledge, skills and attitudes, and the level of knowledge, skills and attitudes they should have within a particular context. The context includes the stage of the course the student is at, as well as the speciality of the practice area they are working in. Regularly assessing a student's learning needs is therefore essential to help you plan relevant learning opportunities and activities. Students are encouraged to identify their own learning needs, and this activity is commonly built into practice assessment documentation. Students are commonly required to identify learning opportunities that are available; identify their own specific learning needs in relation to the placement; make a plan of how these are to be achieved and record progress towards these outcomes.

Once students have identified learning objectives and needs, how these will be achieved requires consideration of learning opportunities. You can help your students identify different aspects of practice learning that will present the learning opportunities needed to develop knowledge, skills and behaviours included in the objectives. Students need to be provided with opportunities to connect existing knowledge with new learning. Placement offers a range of learning opportunities from formal ones as described by your organisation in the initial placement set up and quality audit, through to informal opportunities that you can design and direct. Aim to create learning opportunities from how you learn and believe that students can best learn. Successful students can create opportunities through all sorts of situations. Discussions with the multi-disciplinary team, shadowing colleagues, following a patient/service user as they have care interventions are all common opportunities. In fact, anything that extends knowledge, skills or behaviours and can contribute to developing competence can be learning opportunities. However it's not just about accessing opportunities, but about how students implement learning from these into their practice, or how it guides their development that is important, especially in developing competence. Recording learning from opportunities is vital, to enable the student to establish the value and consolidate the learning. This could be through testimonies or reflections. Such evidence of learning is essential when it comes to making practice assessment decisions. Other common examples include:

- researching conditions, interventions, studying case notes;
- preparing for and presenting care at handovers, meetings;
- visiting related clinical areas;
- talking to carers and families regarding care experiences;
- attending courses within the organisation;
- broadening technical/equipment knowledge;
- working with other colleagues in your area;
- reading specialist journals, text books.

There will be a breadth of learning opportunities for your particular practice area. Thinking about what learning opportunities are currently available or could potentially be available, will help to prepare you for your role as practice supervisor and/or assessor.

Activity 5.5 Leadership and management

Think about your learning needs in relation to your developing role in supporting students in practice. From this, write a minimum of one SMART learning objective for yourself regarding your learning needs. Remember that learning objectives offer a way of breaking down learning into sizeable steps. Once you have completed this task, think about and list the potential learning opportunities in your work area and wider organisation, available to you to help you achieve the outcome

There is no correct answer to this activity, as it depends on your own experience and skills. However, you should talk with your colleagues about your answer. It would be useful to select colleagues who are already practice supervisors and assessors in your area, the learning environment manager, education lead, link lecturer or your line manager. Whilst you are developing your new skills, it is important to network with others and find a role model who will help you achieve this. Referring back to your notes from Activity 5.2 might help you identify colleagues to help you with your developing skills.

Thinking of yourself as a learner with learning needs as in Activity 5.5 can provide you with an opportunity for you to practise your skills in writing learning outcomes. This will then help you to support students with writing learning outcomes. An RCN toolkit published in 2017 provides guidance for mentors of nursing and midwifery students and includes a number of suggestions that should be considered both at the start and during a placement (RCN, 2017a):

- Find out about the student's stage of training.
- Note any previous development needs and past mentor decisions.
- Ask about any specific learning objectives, competence and skills development required in the placement.
- Help the student to form achievable objectives.
- Introduce them to the placement learning opportunities.
- Ask if they need any additional support.
- Identify any specific learning needs/requirement for reasonable adjustments to be made.

Your role as a role model

Practice supervisors and assessors are key role models for pre-registration students (NMC, 2018b; RCN, 2017b). Students will be working closely with, observing and emulating the experienced registrants around them. Role modelling fits with the Social Learning Theory proposed by Albert Bandura (1977, p22) who noted that learning would be *exceedingly laborious, not to mention hazardous, if people had to rely solely on the effects of their own actions to inform them what to do*. Fortunately, most of our behaviour from birth is learnt observationally, through role modelling.

Attributes linked to positive role models include being: approachable; friendly; calm; professional; highly motivated; up to date and competent; empathetic and confidence-inspiring. We can see there are many overlaps with these attributes and the ones required for the practice supervisor/assessor roles listed earlier in this chapter. It is often the case that *good* role models in clinical practice are often unaware that they are seen in this way. Students and other staff recognise these qualities and naturally drift to work with that individual wherever they can. In Scenario 5.1 we can imagine that Mike is an effective role model from some of the attributes Anil has fed back to him, as well as by the way he is often asked by students if they can work with him.

Learning from role models happens through our subconscious, whether or not learning was planned or unplanned. One of the fundamental benefits of role modelling is to help socialise students into the profession and working environment. From their first encounters into the new work area, welcoming and including students and helping them to *belong* is critical to their development. This helps the student to establish the cultural norms. Role modelling helps students to learn the complex professional behaviours that are often too difficult describe. This important role is recognised in the NMC Code (NMC, 2015) as point 20.8 expects all registrants to *act as a role model of professional behaviour for students and newly qualified nurses and midwives to aspire to.*

Although the majority of experiences of role modelling are positive, students can potentially learn undesirable behaviours through this means, and assume that the registrant is always correct and competent. Students might feel that they need to *fit in* and compromise their idealised concept of care delivery. Encouraging students to ask questions of their role models is therefore essential. In addition, equipping students with critical thinking and problem-solving skills can help them to recognise and enjoy good practice. Nursing and midwifery courses are usually designed in a way that ensures students have the opportunity to work with a number of supervisors and assessors. This exposes them to a variety of behaviours and encourages them to identify traits they wish to emulate in their practice as opposed to simply following what their *official mentor* does (Felstead and Springett, 2016).

Your role as a teacher

As well as experience and positive attitude, effective practice supervisors and assessors require additional knowledge and skills related to **pedagogy**. Student nurses and midwives need to be prepared to be highly skilled and knowledgeable. They need to be self-directed, able to work collaboratively or autonomously. As such, diverse student-centred teaching and learning methods are available to us to help to develop these attributes. There are many teaching methods available to support and facilitate learning in the workplace. Chapter 4 explores learning theories and preferred learning styles which empower students with their learning. In this chapter we build on this and Table 5.3 outlines some of the common teaching methods used in clinical practice as well as their advantages and disadvantages. You might already be aware of your preferred methods when you are teaching students, peers or patients/service users/clients in your practice setting. Although these methods have unique differences, they share an adult learning approach in that as a teacher you are facilitative as opposed to instructive. It is important to note that no single best method exists. We are challenged as practice supervisors and assessors to differentiate and adapt our teaching approach to meet individual students' learning needs and styles wherever possible.

Effective teaching methods can engage students in an active learning process and if used well, students are likely to develop their knowledge and skill base. It is important for those involved in educating nurses and midwives to select appropriate teaching methods in order to deliver a high-quality educational experience. In addition, using a range of methods will add to student learning and engagement, as well as develop your repertoire.

Reflective teaching practice

Practice supervisors and assessors will use a wide variety of methods and modes of delivery to facilitate active student learning. Reflective practice is a professional requirement as embedded in the NMC Code (2015) and standards for practice. Our patients/service users/clients wouldn't expect us to work as a nurse or midwife without having subject knowledge and skills, and being familiar with best ways of practising. Equally, our students won't want to be supervised, assessed or taught by someone who doesn't know the subject or the best ways of teaching and learning. Reflective practice encourages us to understand students' needs and abilities in relation to our own abilities. Reflective teachers are more likely to be able to develop reflective students. Chapter 1 of this book introduces reflection and reflective practice in more detail. Activity 5.6 encourages you to reflect on an experience of teaching students or being taught as a student yourself.

Common teaching methods	What are these?	What are the advantages of this method?	What are the disadvantages of this method?
Lectures	This is one of the most basic teaching strategies, using a classroom and a presentation. PowerPoint, Prezi and videos are commonly used to present information. Lectures tend to be less interactive and more teacher led. Online surveys can increase interaction.	Lectures can quickly provide a large amount of information to a large number of students; therefore they are efficient and cost-effective. They are useful to introduce new materials, complex content, models and frameworks.	They can be viewed as boring as they can put the student in a passive, information-receiving role. Students are exposed to information but are not given the opportunity to further process it. The teacher requires effective presentation skills for student engagement.
Seminars	A seminar is a group meeting, usually involving a presentation of some description from a teacher, then some related interactive work. The students should participate at least as actively as the teacher in a seminar.	There are similar advantages to those of a lecture other than seminar groups are smaller, with usually a maximum of 10 students recommended in a practice setting. In addition to introducing new information, the seminar then provides opportunity for deeper learning activities through student interaction and engagement with additional learning activities.	These often work best when students have undertaken some preparation work prior to the seminar, or have relevant experience to offer. They require facilitative skills from the teacher, and engaged, self-directed students.
Tutorials	These are usually a one-to-one session between a teacher and a student where both are equally active in the discussion and presentation of ideas. They are often used in universities and in traditional mentoring relationships in practice.	They are highly individualised for the student. They can be tailored to the student's needs, building on their previous experiences as well as clinical context. They can be useful to support assessment decisions in clinical practice areas. Tutorials don't require specific resources, and can be undertaken anywhere and at any time.	They require facilitative skills from the teacher as well as a good understanding of the students' learning needs. The one-to-one nature of tutorials makes them resource intensive and potentially challenging for some individuals.
Simulation/ High Fidelity Simulation	Simulation attempts to recreate a clinical scenario in an artificial setting. It has been a part of health professional education for decades as it mimics the care environment and allows for direct application of theoretical knowledge and skill demonstration, more than most other methods of teaching.	It provides experiences that help nurses and midwives develop clinical competence in a realistic and safe environment without the potential of harm to patients. This approach utilises the application and integration of knowledge, skills, professional behaviours as well as critical thinking. It can broaden exposure to scenarios, and allows the student time to 'practice'.	Simulation equipment is often expensive to buy/set up and maintain. Even in good simulation training events, it remains 'simulation' and not a 'real experience'. Simulation facilitators have to be well prepared in planning and running simulation events. A debriefing session is critical after any simulation to improve critical thinking and reasoning skills.

Role play	This is an interactive learning technique where students and teacher act out situations and scenarios. Helpful in experiencing the role of another or role expectations. The focus is not on acting but the actions of each 'player'.	Role play is often used to develop skills relating to communication, difficult conversations, professional behaviours and cultural sensitivity scenarios.

They can be spontaneous, not requiring equipment or specific resources. Role play is useful to help practice assessors make decisions or clarify behaviours and judgements of a student. | Not everyone is comfortable with role playing and this might affect performance. In addition, some students might find it hard to take the scenarios seriously. Good facilitation skills are therefore required.

A debriefing session at the end is required to improve critical thinking and reasoning skills. |
| **Guided reflection/ reflective discussions** | Reflection can provide a structure for students to make sense of learning experiences. This ensures that concepts and theories become embedded in practice. | Students can be facilitated to reflect during or immediately after practice experiences about what they have learnt. It is timely, and no additional resources are required.

Students can critically appraise what has been experienced via their practice through reflection. This in turn will support improvement of their ongoing practice.

Reflection can help students recognise how they are professionally developing and areas they are mastering

When reflection involves others, it provides an opportunity to collaborate and share ideas about learning, changes, and new ways of working.

Reflection also opens up an opportunity for open dialogue about a student's performance. | Reflecting critically and sharing this with others can be daunting for students.

Some clinicians report that reflective discussion is more useful than written reflection, which can be time consuming. Also, reflective discussions are not always helpful if the teacher's assessment differs from the student's assessment of their practice.

Reflective practice is more difficult for some students' learning styles than others.

However, all health professions have a requirement for reflective practice so working around some of the disadvantages is of benefit. The facilitator can discuss a requirement for open-mindedness and willingness to listen to others. |

(Continued)

Table 5.3 (Continued)

Common teaching methods	What are these?	What are the advantages of this method?	What are the disadvantages of this method?
Concept mapping	This is a technique to allow students to understand relationships between complex scenarios, cases and conditions, by creating a visual map Mapping is logical, and flexible enough to be revised. Concept maps are sometimes referred to as spider diagrams, mind maps or diagramming.	Concept maps enable students to visualise connections and links, building on ideas they already have, information they know already and experiences they have had. In particular, with clinical cases and patient journeys. They also identify gaps in knowledge the student has, to help them further plan. This technique helps students to analyse, evaluate and critically think about practice and theory. It can enable students to think holistically, understanding elements of care and the patient/service user/client experience. It can motivate students offering learner autonomy	It is important for the teacher to provide feedback on concept maps to ensure students are not muddling complex relationships. This technique works well for visual learners, but may not be so effective for students with other learning styles.
Educational games/ gaming	Educational games are activities that have been specifically designed to help students to learn. They could introduce information about certain conditions, treatments and interventions; or reinforce students' understanding. Some games are designed to develop particular skills, for example leadership or management.	Games can improve student knowledge through reinforcement of information. They are often used in addition to other methods, i.e. following presentation of material at a lecture. Games encourage active learning and engagement. They can make the learning of difficult content more enjoyable. Games can be used for different levels of complexity. At one level this might be a matching game with labels and diagrams. Other games might involve strategy and encourage critical thinking skills. Games provide instant feedback. Games that can be played on mobile devices can make learning more interesting and connect students to a wider network of students.	Games take time and effort to plan and create. Even in their simplest form, they are resource intensive to develop, so consider the reusability of any game you create. If you use existing games, they could be expensive to purchase and for online games, there may be a subscription cost. Some critics of educational gaming suggest they reduce the student's attention span, which then impacts on other learning opportunities.

Debating	Debating refers to a particular type of discussion where two or more people take on opposing positions on a topic or question with the aim of making others accept their position. Students are involved in actively learning about the content to be debated, and given time to research the issue beforehand.	This method allows students to explore and gain insight into other viewpoints. Particularly useful when teaching about a controversial issue. Debaters examine relevant literature, analyse the data, develop solutions and present their ideas clearly and during the debate. Communication and critical thinking skills are developed as well as higher order learning skills such as analysis and evaluation. Debating can also develop professional advocacy skills for students to learn how to defend particular positions.	Debating requires facilitative skills from the teacher as well as adequate preparation time for the students. Debating is not suitable for all types of content, particularly when there are limited options or solutions. The debater's delivery of their argument can be more influential than the message itself. Good facilitation skills are required to emphasise key learning points.
Problem-based learning (PBL)	This is a student-centred approach where students use 'triggers' from a case or scenario to acquire and apply information to the problem. Students learn through the experience of developing their own learning objectives, undertaking self-directed learning, then returning to the teacher to discuss and refine their acquired knowledge.	Teachers can use real patient scenarios, and require students to search for holistic answers. It's a useful method for complex information, for example clinical case management. This approach encourages self-directed learning; clinical judgement; real-world clinical problem-solving skills; working with others and across disciplines and integration of theory and practice. The self-directed nature of PBL promotes the retention of learnt materials.	One common criticism of PBL is that students might not really know what is important for them to learn. This is especially relevant if they have little or no prior experience. PBL requires facilitative skills from the teacher as well as managing the discussion process and giving feedback on the learning. There is also a requirement of time needed for the student to undertake PBL.
Case studies	Case studies usually involve a description of a real-world situation involving a decision made and subsequent challenges and opportunities. Real clinical cases are commonly used, and access to clinical	This is a useful approach in clinical practice as it bridges the gap between theory and practice. This is often an approach clinicians are very familiar with as case studies are reviewed regularly as continuing professional development activities or multi-disciplinary team meetings.	Students might identify issues that conflict with practice or the clinician's own decisions. This will need facilitation and debriefing to help the student make sense of practice or escalate concerns.

(Continued)

Table 5.3 (Continued)

Common teaching methods	What are these?	What are the advantages of this method?	What are the disadvantages of this method?
	records and investigations are made accessible. Case study findings are anonymised and presented to the teacher and/or others.	Case studies provide practice with recognising 'problems', articulating clinical practice decisions and evaluating interventions. This approach also supports students to be self-directed and think professionally whilst learning about practice. It requires no additional resources. Similarly to PBL, case studies develop collaborative skills as well as skills in organising self, researching and presentation.	The case might have too narrow a focus, or if too complex may result in not enough depth about the condition being learnt by the student. There is also a requirement of time needed for the student to undertake a case study. Similarly to other self-directed methods, some students may struggle with what's expected of them with this approach.
'Bedside' teaching	This approach refers to clinical teaching in the presence of the *real* patient/service user/client. The learning interactions occur directly with the registrant, student and patient/service user/client.	This is a useful approach in clinical practice as it requires no additional resources and bridges the gap between theory and practice. This is often an approach clinicians are very familiar with. Students are provided with an opportunity to learn real-world clinical skills, clinical reasoning, communication, empathy and professionalism. It is particularly useful to teach a holistic picture of a condition, treatments and interventions. It should involve all three parties equally – each individual member brings their own value to the learning triad. The student brings condition specific knowledge and the eagerness to learn; the tutor brings depth of knowledge, and willingness to help the student learn; and the patient brings relevant *real* clinical issues that allow the student to learn.	Bedside teaching needs to be student focused, linked to the student's learning requirements and needs. There is a requirement to prepare the patient/service user/carer as to the learning experience. There needs to be a commitment to uninterrupted time for bedside teaching. The teacher needs to prepare to deal with a number of different issues that might arise during the teaching and may require follow up after the teaching has finished.

Table 5.3   Common teaching methods used in clinical practice and their advantages and disadvantages

Activity 5.6   Reflection

Reflect upon a recent teaching and learning experience, and in particular the teaching method used. This could be one that you were involved in delivering to a student, colleague or patient/service user/client. You could also reflect upon an experience where you were on the receiving end of the teaching and learning activity. The prompts here are adapted from the NMC Revalidation Reflective Accounts Form (NMC, 2017a). (You may wish to use this activity towards your NMC revalidation.)

- What was the nature of the teaching and learning activity in your practice?
- What did you learn from the teaching and learning activity?
- How did you change or improve your practice as a result?

There is no correct answer to this activity, as it depends on your own experience and workplace. However, you might have noted a particular teaching method that you would like to explore further.

Read the section 'Teaching and Learning Approaches and Activities' in Chapter 5 of Gravells, A (2017) *Principles and Practices of Teaching and Training: A Guide for Teachers and Trainers in the FE and Skills Sector*, London: Learning Matters. This provides further insight into teaching methods.

Using technology for teaching and learning

Most of us are increasingly using technology in our everyday lives, including for learning activities. Perhaps you reflected on a teaching session involving technology in Activity 5.6? Those of us supporting students should be aiming to understand how students use and interact with technology during their learning experiences. In addition, we need to be mindful of how tomorrow's registrants will engage with electronic health records (EHRs), wearable technologies, big data, data analytics and increased patient technological engagement. More than ever before, we need to support students to be open to technological advancements and challenges that do not yet exist.

Key findings from a research study of undergraduate students and their technology use by Brooks (2016) include:

- students have many devices they use to gather information;
- students have positive attitudes towards the use of technology for learning;
- students find the use of technology important for them to succeed;
- device ownership is higher among students than in the general population;
- the majority of students have a preference towards blended learning, utilising both online and face-to-face experiences.

Technologies that assist students in identifying individual strengths and weaknesses are particularly helpful for nurse and midwifery students. Also useful are smart devices and apps that can offer an opportunity for students to tailor resources to their learning needs as well as learning when they want to and at their own pace.

Scenario 5.2

Mike has noticed that some students in his practice area appear to struggle with understanding the relevant anatomy and physiology related to his speciality. On occasions, he has directed them to books and articles he has found helpful for learning this. He asks around the students in his area about their preferences for accessing learning materials and finds out that the majority of students prefer to look up anatomy and physiology information from internet sources. He reflects upon this and decides to research good sources of internet anatomy and physiology material linked to his practice speciality. He discovers an app that is free to use and interactive. As well as being informative and aimed at health professionals, it also includes interactive diagrams and video clips. There is also a short quiz to test learning, providing instant feedback. He now recommends that students download and use this app to support their anatomy and physiology learning.

Engaging with technology to support your students' learning will help you to provide a good learning experience and meet the needs of diverse students.

Chapter summary

This chapter has introduced you to the key skills and attributes required to be a practice supervisor and/or a practice assessor. It has provided an overview of the purpose, benefits and principles of a collaborative approach to supporting student learning in practice. By completing the activities you have considered your own skills and attributes you bring to this role, as well as identifying colleagues involved in supporting students in your own practice setting. In addition, you have developed your skills in writing SMART objectives, as well as recognising learning needs and associated learning opportunities. Common teaching methods used in clinical practice have been introduced, as well as some advantages and disadvantages to these methods. Through the scenario, we noted how every registrant has a part to play in supporting students' learning in practice.

Activity answers

Activity 5.1: Reflection (p83)

There is no correct answer to this activity, as it depends on your own experience and skills. However, you have probably noticed that you have many of these skills and attributes already.

Thinking about how you have acquired these already will help you to work on any gaps. If you are not sure, seek feedback from your colleagues or students in your workplace. Reviewing your last appraisal feedback might also help.

Activity 5.2: Reflection (p85)

There is no correct answer to this activity, as it depends on your own experience and workplace. However, you have probably noticed that you have many different roles and registrants in your area who are impacting in some way on the students' learning experience. Maybe you have identified roles including: practice supervisors; practice assessors; learning environment managers; educational leads; link lecturers. These roles are introduced in Chapter 1 and you might want to refer to this chapter to further think about the roles you have listed from this activity. You might have listed others in your area that do not have a specific remit for supporting students, but who do this as part of their wider role. Roles will vary greatly between organisations. Your critical thinking in this activity might have resulted in you recognising that there is some overlap as to the features of these roles.

Activity 5.3: Evidence-based practice and research (p86–7)

There is no correct answer to this activity, as it depends on your own experience and workplace. However, you may have noticed some factors or issues for consideration that you have no one responsible for in your workplace. It may be useful to talk about this with your colleagues, perhaps at a staff meeting, or with those in lead educational roles, for example a Learning Environment Manager. You might find it useful to read Chapter 3 of Ellis and Bach's book *Leadership, Management and Team Working in Nursing* (2015), published by Sage/Learning Matters.

Activity 5.4: Critical thinking (p89)

1. Anil's objective is not SMART.

2. A SMART version of Anil's objective would be *by the end of the second week of placement, I will be able to plan and deliver all care required during the shift, to a bay of six patients under indirect supervision from a registrant.* This objective is SMART as it is specific in who is doing this, and what it is; is measurable; is achievable in light of Anil's experience and level of training; is realistic in terms of what he is required to do within his course; and has a time frame to be achieved within the first two weeks of placement. Working with a SMART learning outcome makes it easier for Anil to communicate what he is doing, as well as for Mike to provide support and feedback on his learning and progress.

Further reading

'Teaching and Learning Approaches and Activities', Chapter 5 of Gravells, A. (2017) *Principles and Practices of Teaching and Training: A Guide for Teachers and Trainers in the FE and Skills Sector*, London: Sage/Learning Matters. This provides further insight into teaching methods and using technology for learning. It has many activities and examples to help you further develop skills in this area.

Chapter 3 of Ellis and Bach (2015) *Leadership, Management and Team Working in Nursing*, Teaching Nursing Practice Series, London: Sage/Learning Matters. This book has some great chapters considering staff development and motivation, mentoring, supervising and creating a learning environment. In particular, Chapter 3 considers team working in detail, which is helpful in developing our collaborative approach to student support.

Chapter 6 Curricula and assessment

Standards Framework for Nursing and Midwifery Education. Part 1 of Realising Professionalism: Standards for Education and Training (NMC, 2018d)

This chapter will address the standards in heading **5: Curricula and assessment**.

5.1 Curricula and assessments are designed, developed, delivered and evaluated to ensure that students achieve the proficiencies and outcomes for their approved programme.

The Code: Professional Standards of Practice and Behaviour for Nurses and Midwives (NMC, 2015)

This chapter most closely aligns with the following professional standards.

Prioritise people

1.1 treat people with kindness, respect and compassion.

1.2 make sure you deliver the fundamentals of care effectively.

1.3 avoid making assumptions and recognise diversity and individual choice.

Practise effectively

6.1 make sure that any information or advice given is evidence based, including information relating to using any healthcare products or services.

6.2 maintain the knowledge and skills you need for safe and effective practice.

7.1 use terms that people in your care, colleagues and the public can understand.

8.1 respect the skills, expertise and contributions of your colleagues, referring matters to them when appropriate.

8.2 maintain effective communication with colleagues.

8.4 work with colleagues to evaluate the quality of your work and that of the team.

8.5 work with colleagues to preserve the safety of those receiving care.

8.6   share information to identify and reduce risk.

9   share your skills, knowledge and experience for the benefit of people receiving care and your colleagues (9.1–9.4).

10.1   complete all records at the time or as soon as possible after an event, recording if the notes are written sometime after the event.

11   be accountable for your decisions to delegate tasks and duties to other people (11.1–11.3).

Promote professionalism and trust

20.2   act with honesty and integrity at all times, treating people fairly and without discrimination, bullying or harassment.

20.3   be aware at all times of how your behaviour can affect and influence the behaviour of other people.

20.8   act as a role model of professional behaviour for students and newly qualified nurses and midwives to aspire to.

25.2   support any staff you may be responsible for to follow the Code at all times. They must have the knowledge, skills and competence for safe practice; and understand how to raise any concerns linked to any circumstances where the Code has, or could be, broken.

Chapter aims

After reading this chapter, you will be able to:

- understand what is meant by assessment and competence;
- develop an understanding of key assessment methods;
- articulate the benefits of involving others in assessment decisions;
- understand the purpose, benefits and principles of feedback.

Introduction

Yasmeen is a student approaching the end of her second year and has a number of practice competencies still to achieve. In this chapter we meet her and her practice supervisor, Jan, at the start of Yasmeen's placement. This chapter begins by considering assessment of competence as a fundamental part of a student's curriculum. We then identify common assessment methods and some of the quality issues associated with assessment. We consider the role others have to play in assessment decisions for our students. The chapter concludes by exploring feedback and the implications it has for learning and progression.

Scenario 6.1

Yasmeen is a student nurse on a community placement at the end of her second year. On her first day she meets with her practice supervisor, Jan, to review her placement assessment documentation and set some objectives. She shows Jan the record of proficiencies that she is expected to achieve by the end of Year 2, from her documentation. Jan can see that Yasmeen has a number of gaps still to be *signed off* as *safe practice* in the clinical skills section including: Nutrition and Hydration; Medicines Management; Assisting with Elimination and Infection Prevention and Control. Yasmeen explains that on her previous placements this year, she has had little opportunity to be assessed on these clinical skills and that she would like to focus on these during this placement. She also explains that during her last placement she had to take a number of weeks' leave from the programme as she was the main carer for a close family member who has since died. Jan confides that she too has recently had a family bereavement and sympathises with Yasmeen.

Assessing competence

We regularly hear and use the terms *competencies* and *proficiencies* in healthcare practice, from student assessments to our own revalidation and pay awards process. The NMC uses these terms to describe the skills and the ability to practise safely and effectively without the need for supervision. They also detail that competence must be consistently maintained throughout careers (NMC, 2018a). Safety is the most important principle in the assessment of competence of nursing and midwifery students and the standards reflect this by ensuring that students achieve a baseline level of competence at the time of entry to the register (NMC, 2011; NMC, 2018a). It is these standards that inform the assessment requirements for the students you are working with.

How do we decide if a student is competent or proficient? There are two main approaches to considering competence. The first focuses on tasks and skills and requires the direct observation of performance of these to evidence competence. This approach is referred to as *behaviouristic*. It is sometimes criticised as focusing only on the task being assessed, rather than with what the student might know; their underlying attitudes and knowledge; other attributes; and failing to understand linkages of tasks to other aspects of care. The second approach considers competence in broader clusters of abilities and not so focused on a particular set of tasks. This approach is referred to as *holistic* as competence is viewed as more than the sum of individual competencies. The criticisms of this approach are that individual competencies evidenced through *tasks* are easier to provide evidence towards and transferable to other areas (National Nursing Research Unit, 2009). Activity 6.1 provides you with an opportunity to reflect on which of these approaches is used in your practice setting.

Activity 6.1   Critical thinking

Think about how competencies are assessed in your clinical practice.
Which approach, behaviouristic or holistic, best describes how competence decisions are made?

There is a model answer for this activity at the end of this chapter.

Most students achieve the required competencies during practice, but there are a few who experience difficulty in meeting the required standards, and even with additional support might need to fail. In 2003 the NMC published research by Kathleen Duffy about *failing to fail*, a term used to describe where mentors were passing students whom they thought that they should have failed. This has huge implications for students and the assessors involved, as well as for the nursing profession as a whole and crucially, implications for patient safety. Many more students are reported to *struggle* and reasons for struggling are often complex. Supporting students who are struggling or failing is covered in more detail in Chapter 7.

Achieving competence is an essential component of whether or not the student can progress to the next *part* of the programme. The progression point usually occurs at the end of each year of the programme. As a practice supervisor or assessor, it is important for you to familiarise yourself with the practice assessment documentation used in your workplace as well as the programme plan for your students. Understanding the student's bigger programme as well as their experiences to date is critical in helping you to assess them accurately. You need to be aware of the stage or level they are at and where this particular placement learning experience fits with the wider programme. You can find details about the students' programme and curriculum from the academic staff from the student's AEI who are linked to your practice area. Activity 6.2 will help you to familiarise yourself with the documentation students bring to your practice area.

Activity 6.2 Decision-making

Identify and familiarise yourself with the practice assessment documentation that the students bring to your workplace. You might need to ask colleagues in your work area or from your AEI where you can access a copy of this type of documentation. If you have students from a number of AEIs accessing your workplace for placement, you need to be familiar with multiple assessment documents. Although these might vary from institution to institution, they will all contain a common set of proficiencies required to be met for that part of the student's programme, which will be mapped to the NMC standards (NMC, 2010, 2011, 2018a).

There is a no model answer for this activity as it depends upon your own practice.

Types of assessment

The practice assessment document is the key assessment tool you will use to assess a student's competence and we will now look at assessment in more detail. There are many forms of assessment, but the main types of assessment related to nursing and midwifery programmes are formative and summative assessments. **Formative assessment** refers to assessments for learning, to check on student comprehension, learning needs and learning progress. It provides a *diagnostic* opportunity to identify areas of strengths and weaknesses, from which action plans and learning objectives can be developed. It can also be used to monitor progress. In contrast, **summative assessment** refers to assessments of learning, which are usually more formal assessments to measure specific learning outcomes or criteria at a specific point in the student's learning. This might be at the end of a placement, semester, year or end of programme. Summative assessment examples include: written assignments; examinations; performance indicators, i.e. skills and competencies; portfolios. In Scenario 6.1, Jan might set Yasmeen formative assessments to assess her knowledge and skills about nutrition. This might be a series of questions, from which she might recommend some further reading of guidelines and then observation of Yasmeen undertaking a nutrition assessment. Yasmeen will also complete summative assessment during this placement as she will need to complete the record of achievement in practice. This contains all the necessary evidence to demonstrate she has undertaken the required number of hours, achieved the NMC proficiencies and achieved the proficiencies. Her practice assessment documentation will form part of the summative assessment to pass her second year of the programme, along with the academic summative assessments.

Assessment methods

Students should be able to improve their practice through appropriate assessments. Assessment has to address the level of students' performance, indicating competence and at what level individuals should be judged incompetent. Reviews have found that there is no gold-standard way for measuring clinical competence (National Nursing Research Unit, 2009). Practice assessment documentation will often vary between AEIs. However, there are some consistent elements when helping us to record a decision of competent. Students' placement assessment documentation will include (as a minimum) two levels, or a binary scale. These are *unsafe practice* (i.e. required standard not met) and *safe practice* (i.e. required standard met). Some documentation may include additional criteria to record when the required safe practice level was met beyond *safe* and was either *good* or *excellent*. The criteria to help you judge practice will be mapped to the level of the programme that the student is currently at.

In order to ensure that practitioners are competent, high-quality assessment strategies are needed. There are a variety of methods that can be used to assess a student practically and theoretically. Those traditionally associated with assessing theoretical knowledge include presentations, examinations and assignments. These are not necessarily appropriate for assessing clinical practice. The NMC (2008) advised that the assessment strategy for students should include assessment through direct care, simulation, and other strategies including observation. The NMC requires most assessment of competence to be undertaken through direct observation in practice. Simulation may occur where opportunities to demonstrate competence in practice are limited. Other examples include: **OSCEs**; testimony from others (including service users and carers); student self-assessment; written portfolio of evidence; active participation; interactive reflective discussion; learning contracts; guided study; interviews; service user comments; peer evaluation; collection of data; case studies and team feedback. Common methods of assessing clinical practice are outlined in Table 6.1, along with associated advantages and disadvantages.

Research suggests that students prefer **qualitative approaches to assessment** rather than numerical assessment (Helminen et al., 2014). However, numerical assessment adds objectivity to the process, and transcends any potential language barriers. For example *10 out of 10* is clearer to understand than *a good attempt*. When assessing clinical practice, using a combination of both qualitative and numerical data to inform an assessment decision is helpful. For example, offering verbal (qualitative) feedback as to why you reached a criterion (numerical) decision would be helpful. It is important to note that not all AEIs grade practice and contain numerical assessments. You will need to familiarise yourself with your partner AEI approach to this, and it should be clearly evident in the student's documentation.

Method	Description	Advantages	Disadvantages
Observation	This refers to observing the student undertake skills in practice. Assessors observe to see if the student performs properly. May be *continuous* (over a number of occasions) or *snap-shot* on a singular occasion.	Can be used to assess problem-solving abilities, communication skills, professional attitudes and behaviours if these are modelled during the skill performance. Plans, criteria or checklists used by the assessor during the observation can support the student's development if shared, and aid assessor objectivity. Often, the most effective way to assess student practice, though best used when the assessor uses it with other methods, for example questioning.	Requires the relevant resources and opportunities to be available to undertake the observation of practice – this will need planning. Needs a systematic plan or set of criteria to help the assessor and student focus on what is being observed and assessed. Can cause the student to have *performance anxiety* and then to undertake the skill less proficiently to how they usually do. Being observed may cause the student to perform differently to usual, referred to as the Hawthorne Effect.
Questioning	This refers to asking effective questions related to the practice learning. It enables students' thinking to be clarified, affirmed and revised, extended.	Can be used to assess previous knowledge or skills of the student. Can ascertain the student's ability to reason, critically think, problem solve, synthesise ideas. Can provide feedback for how effective the learning for the student is/has been. It's quick, instant, cost effective and can be undertaken anyplace/anytime.	Requires the assessor to use effective communication skills, understanding when to use closed and open-ended questions. Requires consideration of appropriate questions for level that student is at. Bloom's taxonomy (Su and Osisek, 2011) is helpful for this, where the basic levels of remembering might require questions posed: how; who; why; what; etc. For deeper learning questions might be: *how might you do it differently?*
Quizzes	This refers to a short assessment that can gauge a student's retention and comprehension of a small amount of information. Might be verbal, written or online.	Can function throughout a placement as an informative feedback device allowing both the supervisor/assessor and the students to see where they are excelling or need more focus.	Developing a quiz requires an understanding of the curriculum and what the curriculum expects the student to know, as quizzes should be clearly aligned. Can be time consuming to develop.

		Highly adaptable to different topics, for example: multiple choice questions (useful for recall on guidelines and policy); true or false questions, short answer questions (useful when more understanding required); labelling diagrams (anatomy, equipment); filling in the blank/missing items (symptom management, care planning); matching items (drug interactions, etc.).	
Testimonies	This refers to a formal written statement, about a student's performance, abilities, character or qualities.	Used to authenticate assessment decisions. A patient, service user or carer who has been on the receiving end of care from the student can be one of the most reliable sources of evidence. Equally, a testimony from a colleague, another healthcare professional, can be a fantastic source of evidence for how your student performs when you are not with them, and in a different context.	The assessor must confirm that the information is authentic and current. The person providing the testimony should be informed as to how their testimony will be utilised. Guidance is needed as to how to undertake a testimony.
Simulation/role play	Simulation/role play aims to replicate real patients/ clients, scenarios, or clinical tasks or to mirror real-life situations in clinical settings – with an emphasis on safety	Useful for the development of technical-based skills required for clinical practice, in a safe environment. Enables assessment of infrequent events that the student might not have had the chance to encounter or experience. Can be set up at appropriate times and locations, and repeated as often as necessary. It can be undertaken in-situ with minimal resources. Feedback can be given to students immediately and allow them to understand exactly what went wrong/ right and how they can improve.	Requires access to simulation equipment and other resources. Can be undertaken in amazingly high technology simulation centres, which can be very expensive and require constant updates and maintenance. Not all students/situations are suitable for this It takes effort and preparation to create meaningful experiences.

(Continued)

Table 6.1   (Continued)

Method	Description	Advantages	Disadvantages
Self/peer assessment	Refers to the practice of self/peers grading or providing feedback on clinical skills and performance, based on guidelines or criteria provided by a supervisor/assessor.	Helps students to develop the ability to make judgements, which is both an academic and professional skill. Students gain insight into how peers tackle similar clinical problems. Students learn how to give and receive constructive criticism from peers. Can be an effective use of time and resources, supervisor/assessor acts as a facilitator.	May not be a reliable source of assessment evidence. Peers might not have same understanding of the situation as the registrant. Students may not provide comprehensive feedback to each other. Students may show bias towards friends and avoid low marks for poor work as they might be concerned they may offend peers. Student may lack self-awareness to be able to do this.
Portfolio evidence/reflective discussion	Refers to interpretation of an experience, identifying issues or questions that arise. Involves the creation of hypotheses regarding how to do things better, thereby challenging an individual's practice.	Portfolios allow students to review a broad range of practice and study in detail particular aspects of it. Can analyse strengths and deficiencies as well as reflect on and identify development needs. Through reflection, students learn to scrutinise their own performance and ask what went wrong as well as what went well. An essential professional skill.	Requires clear outcomes to keep reflections and portfolio entries focused. Requires understanding of reflective process, models can help this. Can take time to establish learning and provide an opportunity for feedback. May not be a reliable source of assessment evidence if the student is unable to use reflection or lacks self-awareness.

Table 6.1   Common methods of assessing clinical practice

Assessment quality

A large-scale review of the literature relating to the assessment process of student nurses' and midwives' clinical practice found that it often lacks consistency, varies in quality and is open to the subjective bias of the assessor (Helminen et al., 2016). Clinical assessment commonly relies on observation of the performance of a student by another individual or *observer*, which runs the risk of observer bias. This describes the idea that there is a tendency for an observer to observe what they are expecting or wanting to see. When observing a student, the supervisor or assessor might have some prior knowledge or subjective feelings about the student that might affect their judgements. In Scenario 6.1, Jan and Yasmeen will have spent lots of time together during Yasmeen's placement. They might have spoken socially as they share long car journeys between their case visits and discovered they share some similar interests. When Jan is assessing Yasmeen's clinical skills, it is possible that she might not be able to objectively do this.

The NMC *Standards for Student Supervision and Assessment* (NMC, 2018b) has clearly separated practice learning and supervision from formal independent assessment in an attempt to reduce bias. The standards have achieved this by moving away from the traditional mentor model, where the mentor was responsible for all aspects of practice learning, supervision and assessment. Instead they have prescribed two distinct roles of practice supervisor and practice assessor to replace the mentor role. The practice supervisor will work with the student on a regular basis. The practice assessors will not be working with students on a day-to-day basis, but will have the responsibility for their assessment. Assessors will be expected to interact with practice supervisors, student peers, service users and other people to gain an understanding of the student's performance. In addition, they must also undertake direct observations of student learning in practice. This will be supported by appropriately recording progress and proficiency outcomes in all student practice assessment documentation. If we apply these standards to Scenario 6.1, a colleague of Jan's will be assigned to be the student's practice assessor. This registrant will be responsible for assessing Yasmeen's competencies, taking into account feedback from Jan, thereby reducing observer bias.

Healthcare programmes usually include set assessments at key stages of the programme as well as continuous assessment throughout the programme. Continuous assessment aims to measure competence at varying points in time rather than at one key point. Assessment at key stages is to decide if the student is able to progress to the next stage of the programme (an example might be to progress into the next year).

With all assessments, two issues are important: how and what is being measured. Methods of assessment should depend upon what is being assessed. If we think back to Scenario 6.1, when Yasmeen undertakes an aseptic wound dressing as part of her assessed competencies, her assessor could supplement the evidence she has from the direct observation of her performing of the skill with some questions afterwards, and potentially any feedback from the patient. Validity refers to the quality of the assessment, whether it actually measures what it intends to measure. If Yasmeen is required to be able to *demonstrate an aseptic technique*, using questions alone would not be a valid assessment for this. Using more than one method of assessment will increase the validity. The concept of triangulation of assessment in educational terms describes how an assessor can use several sources of data or evidence, obtained from different sources, to help them make an assessment decision. By using different sources of data, the assessors can verify the data against each other to help them form a more rounded picture of their student's abilities. Applying this to Scenario 6.1, Yasmeen's practice assessor might use a combination of observation, questioning and testimony evidence to help her reach a decision about Yasmeen's competencies. Reliability of assessments refers to the measure providing similar results if used on different occasions and by different assessors. If an assessment provides an accurate measurement of a student's performance, there should be consistency in results. In the scenario, the practice assessor will be using a set of guidelines that the Trust has developed relating to aseptic techniques. Yasmeen will have been made aware of these guidelines early in the placement by Jan and that these would be used to assess her practice. Using guidelines or criteria for assessing practice aids reliability as it objectifies the skill being assessed and removes any variance that individual assessors could have.

Involving others in assessment decisions

The patient, service user or carer voice has become a principal concept in the quality assurance processes of standards for practice, education and training. There is a requirement that programme providers must make it explicit how patients, service users and carers contribute to the assessment process (NMC, 2018b). This recognises and places a value on the expertise that patients, service users and carers bring. This is supported by the *Report of the Mid Staffordshire NHS Foundation Trust Public Inquiry* (Francis, 2013) which recommended a common culture of putting the patient first. In addition, the *Review into the Quality of Care and Treatment Provided by 14 Hospital Trusts in England*

Activity 6.3   Reflection

Think of a time when you have been involved in the assessment of a student in your work area.

- Did you/colleagues use feedback from patients, service users or carers to inform the assessment decision? If so, how was this obtained?
- Thinking about the considerations involved in asking those in care situations for feedback, how could this be improved in your work area?

There is a model answer for this activity at the end of this chapter.

identified the need to listen to the views of patients and engage them in service improvement initiatives (Keogh, 2013). Research has also shown the value in feedback from patients, clients, carers and service users which can help with practice assessment decisions (Helminen et al., 2014). Activity 6.3 will help you consider how to best obtain this type of feedback and how to minimise any potential issues with requesting patient feedback and testimonies.

Activity 6.3 highlights that there are many considerations involved in asking those in vulnerable care situations for feedback. These considerations include individuals potentially feeling: pressured to give feedback; required to be positive; responsible for passing or failing a student; not able to have anonymity; too ill to offer opinion; that any input might affect their future care (Atkinson and Williams, 2011). Patient, service user and carer input into the student assessment process are, however, fundamental and these considerations can be successfully managed by the assessor. Obtaining written feedback and testimonies relating to the student's approach to care, communication, compassion and dignity are invaluable to a robust assessment. If you have an opportunity to develop or revise any documentation, work with relevant stakeholders, for example patients, service users or carers, to ensure the wording and design are appropriate. Remember that consent must be obtained by the practice assessor, not by the student, for any assessment feedback.

The NMC (2018c) states that practice supervisors would not be expected to carry out summative practice assessments or sign off student proficiency; however, they would contribute to the assessment of students by providing feedback to the practice assessor. This will be helped through the use of documenting formative commentary on the student's progress in appropriate learning records such as practice assessment documentation. Feedback from practice supervisors is therefore fundamental to student assessment decisions. Practice supervisors should regularly feed back and update on progress as well as provide testimony evidence towards formal assessments.

Feedback

Receiving feedback is a fundamental part of the learning and improvement process for students. Effective and timely feedback is essential for the student–practice supervisor/assessor relationship in order for the student to learn from their experiences. Feedback has been defined as a process whereby students obtain information about their work in order to appreciate the similarities and differences between the appropriate standards for any given work, and the qualities of the work itself, in order to generate improved work (Boud and Molloy, 2013). A literature review examining published research in this area found that feedback was often viewed as challenging to deliver and varied greatly in quality (Pollock et al., 2015). It can be particularly difficult if you are required to feed back on an area of the students practice that needs improving, and many individuals involved in supporting practice learning reported that they found it much easier to provide positive feedback when things are going well. Activity 6.4 is designed to help you enhance your feedback skills.

Activity 6.4 Reflection

Think back to a time when you gave some feedback to a student. You might have been giving positive feedback or giving feedback to a student who was struggling or failing to achieve.

- How did you do this?
- How was it received?
- How did you determine that the student understood the feedback?
- Would you do anything differently next time?

If you have not yet had any experience of giving feedback to a student, think of a time you have provided feedback to any other individual.

There is no model answer for this activity as it refers to your own experience, but there are some related key points about feedback provided at the end of this chapter.

Activity 6.4 helps you to think about how feedback is being received and reminds us that feedback is a two-way process. You will be able to learn and develop from feedback provided by the students you are working with relating to your supervisory or assessor skills. All feedback should be constructive in helping the receiving individual progress and improve. Constructive feedback does not mean only giving positive feedback or praise. It also means giving negative feedback skilfully so that it is useful. Destructive feedback is unhelpful and describes negative feedback given in an unskilled way that leaves the student feeling bad with nothing to build upon. Constructive feedback must be specific and different to general everyday comments you might use like *that's fine* or *keep practising*, etc. Constructive feedback should include detail on performance in reference to relevant criteria, so the student is clear about their progression.

There are recognised principles and characteristics of *good* and constructive feedback (Duffy, 2013; Boud, 2015; Scott, 2014). An awareness of these can help us develop our feedback style and skills. Good and constructive feedback is:

- specific, focused on behaviour that can be changed, not on perceived attitudes or generalisations;
- accurate, factual and based on observation;
- objective, unbiased and unprejudiced;
- timely, given in good time, as soon as possible after the *event*;
- constructive, about what the individual did well and what they could do better, related to goals so the student is able to *use* the feedback;
- ready to be received, to aid motivation. Timing and location can help, feedback is best given in private;
- well communicated. Use principles of good communication to deliver the feedback, check for understanding.

It can be helpful for us when developing our own feedback skills to recognise constructive feedback in other conversations. Scenario 6.2 is an excerpt from a conversation where Jan provides feedback to Yasmeen following a clinical procedure.

Scenario 6.2

Jan has observed Yasmeen undertaking an aseptic wound dressing on an elderly male patient with a leg ulcer. After Yasmeen has finished the procedure, she provides her with some feedback. Here is an excerpt from their conversation.

Jan: *How did you feel about undertaking the wound dressing today?*

Yasmeen: *Ok I guess. I think I did a good job but I'm not sure if I missed anything?*

Jan: *Are you ready for me to provide you with some feedback?*

Yasmeen: *Yes please.*

Jan: *I will work through the criteria related to this clinical procedure and give you feedback on each stage. You clearly obtained verbal informed consent from the patient and I particularly liked how you repeatedly checked his understanding of the procedure before you got started. You followed the Trust procedure for decontaminating your hands both pre and post the procedure and I noted that you took care to remove your watch and wash your wrists. You prepared your sterile field as we have been practising, and because you were familiar with the equipment, this seemed to help you to keep exposure of the wound to a minimum. You followed the care plan and redressed the wound as the plan required. I could see you had a close look at the wound and old dressing, what were you looking for?*

Yasmeen: *I was looking for any signs of wound infection and checking there wasn't any irritation from the old dressing.*

Jan: *Well done! I thought that might be what you were doing. You maintained asepsis throughout. I thought you managed that very well, especially as the patient tried to wriggle his leg at one point, but you were quick to notice and explain why you needed him to keep still. One criterion that you didn't fully meet was maintaining the patient's comfort and dignity throughout the procedure. Although you started the procedure by ensuring he was comfortable, you didn't seem to notice your patient's body language during the procedure. At one point he looked really uncomfortable. Did you notice this?*

Yasmeen: *I think I was too busy focusing on getting the skill right that I forgot to keep checking on his comfort. I will make sure next time that I regularly ask the patient how they are and try and be more observant of their body language.*

(Continued)

(Continued)

Jan: *Yes that would be good. I appreciate there is a lot to focus on when developing your new skills. Try and keep open communication channels throughout the procedure and you will quickly be aware if your patient is uncomfortable. I think in this instance, explaining that you were removing a dressing and it could feel uncomfortable for a few minutes, would have really helped with this. Have I been clear that this one criterion was not fully met, which means you will need to be assessed again against this proficiency?*

Yasmeen: *Yes, I understand.*

Jan: *OK. To continue, I think your documentation of the procedure is clear and detailed and I was especially impressed with your detailed description of the wound.*

Activity 6.5   Evidence-based practice and research

Using your knowledge of principles and characteristics of constructive feedback, read through Scenario 6.2 and think about the conversation between Jan and Yasmeen.

- Does Jan provide Yasmeen with constructive feedback?
- Find examples from the conversation to support your answer.

There is a model answer at the end of this chapter.

Constructive feedback can: promote improvement and development; sustain and increase motivation; increase confidence and self-esteem; increase competence and improve quality of care; promote open communication channels and create a feedback-friendly culture across the wider team, which helps teams improve (Boud, 2015). These benefits are fundamental for the student, but are also noted as being beneficial for the supervisor or assessor who is providing the feedback. If we consider Jan's feedback to Yasmeen in Scenario 6.2, we can see that she largely covered the principles and characteristics of constructive feedback.

Feedback models

Models can provide a structure to the feedback process and are particularly useful when we are developing and refining our skills as supervisors and assessors. There are lots of different feedback models available, and you might find that one particular one works better for your own communication style and your students. Table 6.2 summarises four commonly used models or approaches to feedback in clinical practice.

Feedback model/ approach	Description	Uses
The feedback sandwich	This model consists of three parts where you make positive statements, discuss areas for improvement, and then finish with more positive statements.	This aims to minimise the potential for any detrimental effect of discussing the *negative* aspect
The stop – start – continue	This model consists of three parts where you discuss with your student what they feel they should stop doing; what they feel they should start doing and what they wish to continue doing.	This aims to give the feedback some structure, ensuring the negative part is addressed, but acknowledging the positives to *carry on*
The situation – behaviour – impact	This approach consists of three stages where you begin with defining the situation the feedback refers to; next define the specific behaviours you want to address and end by describing how those behaviours affected you or others.	This allows the student to reflect on their actions while understanding specifically what you are commenting on and why, as well as think about what they need to change.
Pendleton's model of feedback	This model has several stages: 1. Check the student is ready for feedback. 2. The student gives a background to the event/procedure that is being assessed. 3. The student states what was done well. 4. The supervisor/assessor(s) state what was done well. 5. The student states what could be improved. 6. The supervisor/assessor(s) state how it could be improved. 7. An action plan for improvement is made, in partnership between student and supervisor/assessor.	This approach encourages the student to identify areas of improvement, which are then followed by discussion with the supervisor/assessor

Table 6.2 Commonly used feedback models in clinical practice

There are many different models of feedback, which is really helpful as you can find one that best suits you. You might find that you adapt a model to better *fit* your individual style. Being aware of which approach or model you use can be helpful in developing your skills as well as checking that you work through the stages fully. Activity 6.6 provides an opportunity to explore your feedback style a little further.

Activity 6.6   Reflection

Revisit the experience or event you identified in Activity 6.3.

- Did you use a model to structure your feedback? If so which one?
- Do you have a preference towards any of the models outlined in Table 6.2? Now think about how you would have delivered the feedback using the preferred model.

There is no model answer as this activity relates to your experiences. However components of feedback models are further outlined at the end of this chapter.

You may have noted from undertaking Activity 6.6 that you use different feedback styles or models depending upon the type of feedback you are giving. Feedback can sometimes be difficult to give and receive, especially if your student is underperforming. Remember that constructive feedback should always be given in a way that supports professional development. Creating a feedback culture in your workplace means that you support and encourage all kinds of feedback, for colleagues as well as students. Feedback for positive behaviours and practice often gets neglected and forgotten, and you can start to practise this in your own practice setting. Encouraging all types of feedback results in it becoming ultimately easier when you need to give and receive negative feedback.

Chapter summary

This chapter has introduced you to the key concepts of assessment and feedback. It has provided an overview of assessment methods and quality issues relating to assessment. By completing the activities you will have considered the practice assessment documentation that students bring with them to your practice area and started to familiarise yourself with the students' programmes and curricula. You will have reflected upon how you use patient/service user or carer feedback as assessment evidence, the benefits of this and potential issues associated with this. You will have also reflected upon your feedback style and the importance of constructive feedback for learning and progression. Through the scenarios, we noted how proficiencies could be assessed as well as the principles of good feedback. With an increased focus on students working with a range of practice supervisors, we considered how others can effectively support assessment decisions.

Activity answers

Activity 6.1: Critical thinking (p105)

There is no correct answer to this activity, as it depends on your practice area and the approach of the AEIs you work with. However, you have probably noticed that the focus is on tasks and direct observation that are consistent with the behaviouristic approach. Although this approach has its critics, it is useful, especially in professions such as nursing and midwifery, which have many tasks and observable behaviours. This is because individual tasks are easily visible, so the assessment document can be used by multiple assessors while the student moves through the programme to different placements.

Activity 6.3: Reflection (p112)

There is no correct answer to this activity, as it depends on your experience and practice setting. However, you may have already, or may consider developing, a template to use to obtain student feedback or testimonies. Feedback could be in the form of a short questionnaire or set of cue questions. You might include a scale for individuals to *rate* a professional behaviour if this is to be assessed. Templates for testimonies could include prompts for areas you would like feedback on. Information about using the templates would be useful, reminding individuals of what this is for, how it will be used, what is required and rights to anonymity or to be able to refuse to undertake this without any impact upon their care.

Activity 6.4: Reflection (p114)

There is no answer for this activity as it relates to your experiences; however, you might find it useful to read the article by David Boud (2015) Feedback: ensuring that it leads to enhanced learning. *The Clinical Teacher*, 12(1), pp3–7. He summarises with the following key points about feedback:

- Learning involves bridging the gap between desired and actual performance.
- Feedback comments must primarily be judged on their effects on learning and performance.
- It is necessary to look beyond the immediate task: acts of assessment must be designed to leave students better equipped to learn further.
- Learners need to develop a view about what constitutes quality work if they are to demonstrate it for themselves.
- Feedback is not a unilateral act by tutors or trainers, but is a set of interlinked activities.
- Students need always to be positioned by tutors and other staff as pro-active learners who can initiate feedback-seeking behaviour.
- Knowledge of the desires and expectations of the student is needed for effective input.
- Effective learning requires dialogue.
- The overriding purpose of feedback is the refinement of the student's capacity to use information to judge themselves in similar situations.
- Inputs from tutors are important as they can open up or close down learning possibilities.

Activity 6.5: Evidence-based practice and research (p116)

Yes, Jan does provide Yasmeen with constructive feedback.

The table highlights some of the evidence you might have noted from Scenario 6.2.

Principles and characteristics of good feedback	Evidence from Jan's feedback to Yasmeen
Specific	Jan provides specific and detailed feedback about a particular care episode.
Accurate	Jan has observed the care episode and asks questions to Yasmeen during the feedback to clarify any area she is unsure of.
Objective	Jan uses the criteria from Yasmeen's skills documentation and Trust's guidelines to structure the feedback, and judge performance.
Timely	Jan provides feedback in a timely way, soon after the care episode and away from the patient/carer or any colleagues.
Constructive	Feedback is specific and focuses on the care episode; where criteria not met, suggestions for ways to develop practice are offered.
Ready to be received	Jan checks that Yasmeen is ready to receive feedback about this event.
Well communicated	Jan uses appropriate questioning, clear language related to the event, checks for understanding.

Activity 6.6: Reflection (p118)

There is no answer for this activity as it relates to your experiences; however, whichever model you choose to use, or indeed adapt to work best for you, there are four general components to any model or approach you take. Four general characteristics for feedback models are suggested by Askew and Lodge (2000) and these summarise nicely the components of any good feedback:

1. Involve students in conversation about learning which raises their awareness of quality performance.

2. Facilitate feedback processes through which students are encouraged and motivated to monitor and evaluate their own learning.

3. Enhance student capacities for lifelong learning by supporting their development of skills for goal-setting and action planning for learning.

4. Design (formative) assessment tasks in which feedback from varied sources is encouraged, generated, processed and used to enhance their performance.

Further reading

Pollock, CHF, Rice, AM, McMillan, A (2015) *Mentors' and Students' Perspectives on Feedback in Practice Assessment: A Literature Review.* NHS Education for Scotland. This review provides some interesting insights into feedback and its role in practice assessment. The findings section explores how we can seek and use feedback from others in helping support assessment decisions.

Su, WM and Osisek, PJ (2011) The revised Bloom's Taxonomy: Implications for educating nurses. *The Journal of Continuing Education in Nursing,* 42(7): 321–27. This article highlights the usefulness of Bloom's Taxonomy for registrants involved in education and in particular how it can be used to help develop learning objectives at an appropriate level for the student's learning.

Chapter 7 — Students in difficulty

(Continued)

8.2   maintain effective communication with colleagues.

8.4   work with colleagues to evaluate the quality of your work and that of the team.

8.5   work with colleagues to preserve the safety of those receiving care.

8.6   share information to identify and reduce risk.

8.7   be supportive of colleagues who are encountering health or performance problems. However, this support must never compromise or be at the expense of patient or public safety.

9   share your skills, knowledge and experience for the benefit of people receiving care and your colleagues (9.1–9.4).

10.1   complete all records at the time or as soon as possible after an event, recording if the notes are written sometime after the event.

10.2   identify any risks or problems that have arisen and the steps taken to deal with them, so that colleagues who use the records have all the information they need.

11   be accountable for your decisions to delegate tasks and duties to other people (11.1–11.3).

Preserve safety

13.3   ask for help from a suitably qualified and experienced healthcare professional to carry out any action or procedure that is beyond the limits of your competence.

13.5   complete the necessary training before carrying out a new role.

Promote professionalism and trust

20.1   keep to and uphold the standards and values set out in the Code.

20.2   act with honesty and integrity at all times, treating people fairly and without discrimination, bullying or harassment.

20.   uphold the reputation of your profession at all times (20.1–20.10).

25.2   support any staff you may be responsible for to follow the Code at all times. They must have the knowledge, skills and competence for safe practice; and understand how to raise any concerns linked to any circumstances where the Code has, or could be, broken.

Chapter aims

After reading this chapter, you will be able to:

*   recognise the signs of and effects of stress on students in difficulty;
*   understand how to support a student in difficulty using Egan's Skilled Helper model;

- articulate the indicators of a student failing summative practice assessments;
- understand how to use the assessment process to manage a failing student and recognise when and where to seek support for your student and yourself.

Introduction

Most students will complete their placement without too many issues arising or causes for concern. However, occasionally a student might work in a way that is professionally undesirable or that constitutes unacceptable professional conduct. When this impacts upon practice assessment outcomes and the student is clearly failing, there is usually an established process to follow and support mechanisms to access, to help you manage this. However, the student might have behaviours we find professionally difficult, yet is still able to progress through the programme as their assessments don't include any judgement in relation to this. This sort of behaviour usually accounts for a student who is *in difficulty*. Both students in difficulty and failing students present a complex and challenging situation for their practice assessor and supervisors.

In this chapter we will meet Jez who is a first-year student midway through his first placement. His practice supervisor, Kate, has been working most days with Jez, but is concerned about his progress towards achieving his placement outcomes. We will explore some of the signs and effects of stress on students in difficulty, as well as a useful model to help you support students. We will also examine issues around failing students including indicators of failing and the processes involved to manage and support you and your student with this.

Effects of being *in difficulty*

What happens when our students are failing to meet their objectives during their clinical placement? Students might be struggling and *in difficulty* – and we can help as their practice supervisors or assessors. The term *in difficulty* in this context is defined by Health Education England (HEE) (2015) as when a student has *a problem(s) in their education, training, conduct or health, that affects, or is likely to affect significantly, patient safety, team-working, educational progress or their well-being*. It is a term commonly used by health professionals, particularly in medicine and dentistry. It is used to explore students' situations, and also situations registered practitioners might find themselves in at various points of their careers.

We can start by considering how we might recognise this *in difficulty* behaviour, and consider some of the causes for this. We all vary in our capacity for self-regulation of our emotions and this is further compounded by the particular context and physical and psychological state we happen to be in. The emotions involved when a student is struggling could manifest themselves as anger, fear, hostility and disappointment. This might result in a display of difficult behaviours, for example rudeness; hostility; impatience and avoidance. Findings from research studies show that in this situation, the possibility for further errors increases whilst the individual's overall confidence levels drop. In addition, the interpersonal relationship between the struggling student and others deteriorates, as the frustration between themselves and their supervisors/ assessors builds. This is compounded as more people become aware and involved in the situation (Evans and Brown, 2017), for example academics from the student's course. All these factors add to the student's rising stress levels. In Scenario 7.1 we consider some of the signs and behaviours a student in difficulty might display.

Scenario 7.1

This scenario outlines a conversation between Kate, a practice supervisor, and Jez, a first-year student. Jez is halfway through his first placement, and he has been working most of the previous four weeks with Kate. At the start of the week, Kate discussed with Jez at his midpoint interview how she was concerned with his progression towards his placement outcomes. Today Kate takes Jez to a quiet area before they start their shift together to talk more about this, based on events from the previous day. The conversation outlines some of the behaviours a struggling student might be displaying.

Kate: *Do you feel like you've made any more progress towards your outcomes since we spoke last week?*

Jez: *I thought I was until I totally messed up with Mr Davidovic's personal care yesterday. After that it's all gone downhill, I just can't seem to get anything right.*

Kate: *I know that you didn't help him to get washed and dressed in time for his tests as we had planned, but later that day once I'd helped him, he was happy enough with the care he'd received.*

Jez: *That's good to hear!*

Kate: *I was surprised you weren't around to help me with his care, in fact I didn't see you for the rest of the shift yesterday. What were you doing?*

Jez: *(tearful) I'll never be able to do it like you. I didn't think Mr Davidovic would want me anywhere near him after I messed up with getting him ready on time. I think he'll feel better if I'm not involved in his care anymore.*

> Kate: So you just left him and our other patients?
>
> Jez: I thought it better if I went to the day room and looked through those folders you showed me from the office, the ones full of information about treatment procedures.
>
> Kate: Really Jez, that wasn't a good time to be reading about treatments, you left me with lots to do! Today I'd like you to work with Mr Davidovic again; you can start by helping him with his personal care.
>
> Jez: (looks uncomfortable, sighs and walks towards the patient's room)

In Scenario 7.1, we can sense the rising frustration for both parties through the developing conversation. Jez's confidence in his ability to undertake care for Mr Davidovic is low. This is causing him to avoid direct caring opportunities. Kate may be asking Jez to work with Mr Davidovic again as she thinks this will help him confront his anxieties. However, this seems to have resulted in Jez's stress levels rising as he is now in an *uncomfortable* position, and could potentially put the patient's safety and wellbeing at risk.

Recognising students in difficulty

Professional courses like nursing and midwifery require students to have clinical knowledge, skills and attitudes embedded throughout the course. A student in difficulty might be able to meet their placement outcomes as they have the relevant skills and knowledge, but may be struggling with the less tangible development of a *good* professional attitude. Undesirable attitudes are often the hardest aspect for practice supervisors and assessors to address as they are difficult to objectify. The student might seem unmotivated and disinterested, struggling to engage with patients, yourself or the wider team. They might have poor timekeeping, undesirable ways of communicating, or an unsuitable dress code. They could appear anxious or fearful, and as if they are not enjoying the placement. Looking at Scenario 7.1, it is not clear whether it's a skill, knowledge or attitude deficit Jez has or whether there is some other interpersonal difficulty.

It might be that your student is failing to meet their practice outcomes and that you have a clear and tangible measure that they are in difficulty. This often happens if a student is struggling or failing with a particular skill, competence or a technique that is professionally required. If this is the case, you might try further simulation of the assessment task with your student. This could involve role play; simulation aids, for example human mannequins; or further demonstration from yourself or colleagues. In Scenario 7.1 Jez might benefit from observing Kate provide more direct care episodes with patients, before being asked to undertake this again on his own. Further exposure to the situation, more time or supported further attempts can really make a difference.

Chapter 4 highlights different learning styles that can help us to understand behaviours. Sometimes students have difficulty transitioning learning from the classroom into the clinical environment. Simulation can bridge this type of difficulty, and you can facilitate this by providing a safe environment to *practise* the desired skill or behaviour before undertaking it for real. Skills and proficiencies from a practice assessment document often lend themselves to this. Chapter 5 of this book outlines different teaching methods to further encourage student engagement.

There are many stressors involved in being a student, and indeed as a registered health professional, and there is evidence to suggest that some personality characteristics can increase an individual's risk of becoming distressed during placement (Sonnak and Towell, 2001). One of these is imposter syndrome (IS), which is a behaviour characterised by intense feelings of fraudulence when achieving success. This characteristic is commonly linked to students and health professionals. Workplace stress and the IS, and their role in causing some students to get in difficulty, are explored in more detail in this chapter.

Workplace stress

Stress is a part of everyday life, and can be very useful. However, some ways in which we respond to stress can be unhelpful and when experienced over a prolonged period stress can cause us to have physical and psychological problems. NHS Choices (2017) describes stress as *the feeling of being under too much mental or emotional pressure*. When we are no longer able to cope with the pressures we are faced with, this turns into stress, which then impacts how we are able to think, act and cope.

When we are in a stress state or *stressed*, our body is preparing for imminent action, which is known as the *flight or fight response, also referred to as an acute stress response* or *hyper-arousal*. More recently, experts have added *freeze* to the *flight or fight response* to describe a third survival instinct to keep perfectly still, for example like a rabbit might *freeze* when caught in the headlights. This stress state helps the body prepare for impending action by stopping the body's longer-term functions, for example the immune system, by triggering a surge of hormones. Throughout evolution, this has been central to survival for species. It provides energy to escape from danger, or energy to remain and fight. Once the threat has passed, our stress hormone levels soon return to a normal level. However, when this state is prolonged, stress hormones remain at high levels in the body and can lead to health problems.

Your student might be experiencing problems in their personal life, which is affecting their performance at work. This might include loneliness, relationship problems, financial difficulties and problems with mental or physical health. Being in a stressed state is not always recognisable by the person experiencing it. Therefore, it becomes essential for us to recognise potential stress signs in ourselves, students and colleagues around us. Table 7.1 outlines some of the common stress signs, symptoms and behaviours (Health and Safety Executive, no date).

Emotional symptoms	Mental symptoms	Changes in usual behaviours
• Negative or depressive feelings • Disappointment with yourself • Increased emotional reactions – more tearful or sensitive or aggressive • Loneliness, withdrawing from others • Loss of motivation, commitment and confidence • Mood swings	• Confusion • Indecision • Inability to concentrate • Poor memory • Lack of clarity • Lack of ability to prioritise	• Changes in eating habits • Increased smoking, drinking or drug taking activity *to cope* • Mood swings affecting your behaviour • Changes in sleep patterns • Twitchy or nervous behaviour • Changes in attendance such as avoidance, arriving later or taking more time off

Table 7.1   Common stress signs, symptoms and behaviours

There are many stressors involved in being a student, and indeed as a registered health professional. You might recognise some of the emotional and mental symptoms or changes from normal behaviour outlined in Table 7.1 in yourself and others around you. Activity 7.1 offers you an opportunity to reflect on your experiences to date and/ or Scenario 7.1, and identify stress signs, symptoms and behaviours in students.

Activity 7.1   Critical thinking

Think about a student you have previously worked with who was in difficulty. Now look at the common stress signs, symptoms and behaviours summarised in Table 7.1.

- Did the student you have identified display any of these?
- If so, did you find these difficult to handle? How did you respond?

If you have not yet worked with a student who has been in difficulty, use Scenario 7.1 and the information we have about Jez to answer the questions.

There is no correct answer to this activity if it relates to your own experiences. If you have considered Jez's stress signs, symptoms and behaviours from Scenario 7.1, there is a model answer at the end of this chapter.

If you have experience of working with students in difficulty, you might have noted in Activity 7.1 some or all of the stress signs, symptoms and behaviours outlined. The NHS Choices (2017) website offers many valuable activities and exercises for dealing with stress in the workplace and is a good resource for you to use. You might want to direct your students to using this resource, or use it yourself to help you look after your own wellbeing. Further information about looking after your mental wellbeing is provided in Chapter 8.

Stress and the imposter syndrome

Research studies link some personality characteristics with an increased risk of becoming stressed and/or distressed during placement. This, in turn, increases the individual's risk of being *in difficulty*. The characteristics commonly linked to workplace stress is imposter syndrome (IS). IS describes a psychological pattern where an individual has a fear of being exposed as a *fraud* as they have internal doubts about their achievements. It often manifests itself as feelings of self-doubt, fear that an individual's true abilities will be found out and that other people have an over-inflated perception of that individual's abilities (Jarrett, 2010). Students who experience IS believe they have somehow 'fooled' people into believing they are more intelligent and competent than they really are. They often believe they don't deserve success and that they have somehow been lucky *to get away with it* up to this point. A large-scale research study by Christensen et al. (2016) examining IS in nursing students worldwide found younger students and those who had less support in their home life exhibited a higher proportion of imposter-type feelings. They also found that IS manifests itself in times of increased accountability and responsibility, for example during placement and assessment periods.

You might recognise IS in your student if they repeatedly express feelings of self-doubt by saying *I'm not as good as you think I am* or have difficulty taking credit for what they have achieved by saying *I don't deserve to pass this*. They might be frustrated and feel unable to meet their self-set standards if they are a perfectionist and unable to accept anything other than the very high level of performance they have set for themselves. The student could ask of you *I'll never be as good as you so why should I try?* An IS personality trait often leads a student to lack in confidence and have an exaggerated fear of making mistakes. In Scenario 7.1, Jez could be experiencing these feelings as he states *I didn't think he'd want me anywhere near him so I kept away. I'll never be able to do it like you. I think he'll feel better if I'm not involved in his care.*

Some ways in which we can support students to overcome IS and therefore reduce some of their workplace stress, is through assessment and feedback. Research studies have found that IS can be reduced if students are allowed to fail and face disappointment. For example, we could provide practice for tasks (formative), giving students multiple opportunities to fail without it being in a high risk situation (summative) and having repercussions. This develops the student's ability to learn from the failing experience. An example of this could be learning to better receive feedback or learning to reflect on one's own practice. Another suggestion is to discourage students in comparing their own performance to others. Instead, they should be comparing their performance to examples of their own earlier performances. If we apply these suggestions to Scenario 7.1, Kate could provide Jez with additional opportunities for direct patient care. Kate could then provide feedback on each of these opportunities. Chapter 5 explores feedback in more detail. Kate could also ask Jez to think about other care episodes he has been part of and recognise any development from these. Most importantly, students with IS need to be reminded that they are still developing in their careers, which makes it difficult to actually be an *imposter* (Chapman, 2017).

Coping mechanisms for students in difficulty

Students who are in difficulty might employ various coping mechanisms to help them manage the situation that they find themselves in (Steinert, 2008). If as practice supervisors and assessors we can recognise these, we can begin to support our students by helping them to understand that there is an underlying issue that needs addressing (Whitbourne, 2011; Kramer, 2010). Perhaps the student is in denial and makes excuses for their undesirable behaviour, refusing to acknowledge that it exists. Repression involves completely forgetting the experience or event all together. The student might use displacement tactics, and take on more and more work taking them away from the situation they are finding stressful. Alternatively, the student could transfer their emotions from the situation or person who is the target of their frustration, to someone or something else entirely different. They might avoid working with you, in an attempt to further delay you investigating any issues. Another means of coping is reaction formation, where the student becomes angry and frustrated, blaming everyone else for the situation they find themselves in and losing any objectivity.

A common mechanism used by health professionals to cope with tense and stressful situations is humour. You might notice yourself or others around you looking at a funny aspect of a stressful event or situation, which will then help us to endure it. Other defence mechanisms that help individuals cope include intellectualisation, projection and sublimation. A student might reduce their anxiety by thinking about the situation in what seems a cold or detached way. This is referred to as intellectualisation. An example might be that the student who is failing a professional behaviour might focus on learning everything about that behaviour; distancing them self from any actions or behaviour they need to work upon. Projection involves turning our own undesirable attitudes or behaviours and ascribing them to others around us. An example could be if you are addressing poor time keeping with a student who then starts to accuse you of the same behaviour, with little or no evidence. Sublimation describes how an individual can convert undesirable behaviours into more socially acceptable ones. An example might be taking up boxing as a hobby to vent frustrations.

Findings from various research studies have found that registrants at any levels of experience cope with the stresses of work by using psychological defence mechanisms (Williams, 2013; Martins et al., 2014). We might recognise some of these behaviours in ourselves and colleagues as well as in the students working with us. Tillett (2003) undertook research to explore the psychopathology of helping professionals. He found that under extreme work pressure, professional exhaustion and burnout, individuals revert to the use of more substantial and primitive defences, for example denial. The danger arises when individuals become isolated, unable or possibly even unwilling, to compare their perceptions with those of peers and colleagues. The symptoms associated with professional exhaustion or burnout are summarised in Table 7.2. It is helpful to be able to recognise these symptoms to be able to trigger support.

Emotional	Cognitive	Behavioural	Physical
Loss of humour (or excessive use of black humour)	Poor concentration	Work avoidance (absenteeism, clock-watching, etc.)	Tiredness, lethargy
Irritability/resentment/bitterness	Rigidity/resistance to change	Diminished personal contact with clients/colleagues	Sleep disorders
Persistent mood of depression	Suspicion/mistrust	Stereotyped/inflexible behaviour	Increased minor illnesses (e.g. headache, backache)
Feelings of failure/guilt/blame	Stereotyping	Habitual lateness	
Apathy/low energy	Objectification/distancing	Acting out (alcohol/drugs/affairs/shoplifting, etc.)	
	Ruminations (of leaving, revenge, etc.)		

Table 7.2 Symptoms associated with extreme work pressure, professional exhaustion or burnout

Activity 7.2   Reflection

Think about the student you identified in Activity 7.1.

- Did the student you have identified display any of the coping mechanisms outlined in this chapter?
- If so, how did you/others respond?

There is no correct answer to this activity as it relates to your own experiences.

Some of the symptoms outlined in Table 7.2 are relatively common, transient and short lived. Perhaps you noticed this from completing Activity 7.2? Supporting individuals out of difficulty can help, and how you can do this is explored next. However, it is important to note that the most serious dysfunction found in health professionals results from the sustained use of these defence mechanisms combined with professional isolation (Tillett, 2003). An extreme form of this can be seen in registrants who covertly damage patients in their care. Examples of these very extreme cases include the doctor Harold Shipman and the nurse Beverley Allitt who are both convicted serial killers. With their colleagues they displayed very little evidence of any psychiatric disorder. Their professional isolation and lone working hid their major personality disturbances from their colleagues. Their actions were often overlooked or ignored by others who were reluctant to recognise or believe any warning signs. Thankfully, these types of individuals are very rare.

Supporting the student in difficulty

The aim of support is to move the student out of the *difficulty* that if persists, is likely to lead the student to fail. Supportive supervision can really help. This involves: effective communication; a trusting relationship, constructive feedback and choices of learning and assessment methods. Changing or modifying attitudes requires an individual to work on often deep-rooted subconscious beliefs and values, so it requires a lot of effort. Motivation for change must come from the individual student themselves.

There are many models that can be used in a *helping* relationship. One that is particularly useful for students in difficulty is Egan's Skilled Helper model. Traditional approaches to mentoring, coaching and supervision position the *helper* as the expert who identifies what the *problem* is and any subsequent solutions. The student then receives instruction about what to do, with the underpinning philosophy being that knowledge will lead to a change in behaviour. However, this puts the student in a passive position, and rarely results in change behaviour. Research relating to helping students out of difficulty supports the use of an individual-centred model such as Egan's (Newnham-Kanas et al., 2010). This approach acknowledges the reasons for *struggling* or being *in difficulty* are often complex and multi-faceted. It also acknowledges that the student needs to be driving any changes required. Egan's model positions the student as the expert, who if supported, can identify their own issues and goals. The supervisor or assessor facilitates the process, providing cues for action and reinforcing positive behaviour. This, in turn, results in the student developing skills of self-management as well as resilience. Even when a student is not in difficulty, you might find using elements of this model useful to motivate engagement. Equally, you might find the model helpful working with colleagues who are in difficulty.

Using Egan's Skilled Helper model with a student in difficulty

Egan's Skilled Helper model is also used in Chapter 8. It is particularly useful here as it is concise, offers a staged approach and provides structure and guidance for those in supporting roles. It is recognised as being particularly helpful where there is a goal of long-lasting change required. The model has three stages, which can be summarised as: what is going on; what does the individual want instead and how can the individual achieve what they want (Egan, 2013)? Let's consider how we can apply the three stages of Egan's model to the characters in Scenario 7.2.

Scenario 7.2

Kate is familiar with Egan's Skilled Helper model and has used this before. Prior to arranging a meeting with Jez, Kate reflects upon how she has used this model previously with students. She writes herself a plan of how she might use the model with Jez, and notes down prompts for her to use at each stage. She plans for Jez to be doing most of the talking in the meeting, and she finds it helpful to make some notes to remind her how to ask open-ended questions. Kate's preparation notes are as follows.

> *First actions* – *Arrange a first meeting with Jez, check our schedules and ensure we can have 1 hour uninterrupted. Arrange a suitable room, let Jez know these details.*
>
> *During the meeting* – *Work through Egan's 3 stage model (although we might need a series of meetings for this).*
>
> *Stage 1: Telling the story*
>
> *Aim of the stage* – *To provide a safe place for the student to tell their story and uncover the current scenario.*
>
> *Notes* – *Involves creating a space to hear and understand Jez's story in his own words. I can help him to see the wider picture and any other perspectives, finding a point to be able to move forwards. I should be aiming to provide hope.*
>
> *1a The story* – *encourage Jez to talk about what's really going on. Use effective active listening skills including open questions, summarising, paraphrasing and reflecting. Useful questions:* How did you feel...?; What were you thinking when... *and* What else is there about that...
>
> *1b Blind spots* – *Help Jez to find out what's really going on, uncovering any gaps in his assessment of the situation. Any impact of his behaviour on others, strengths, etc. I should be challenging, helping Jez to recognise any discrepancies, distortions or if he's not fully aware. Useful questions:* How might others see this...?; Is there any other way of looking at this ...?; *or* What about all of this, is an issue for you?
>
> *1c Leverage* – *Focus and move forward. Help move Jez from being stuck to moving forwards and having hope. Help him to choose an area he has energy to work on to start to move forwards that will make a difference and be of benefit to him. Useful questions:* What in all this is the most important to you?; What is manageable? *and* What might make the most difference to...?

Stage 2: The preferred picture

Aim of the stage – To help the student find what they want instead.

Notes – Ensure Jez reflects upon what he really wants from this, instead of jumping straight into a solution to what he's identified as an issue in stage 1.

2a Possibilities – Help Jez to brainstorm his ideal scenario, note down brainstorm ideas. Make sure I am non-judgemental and don't add my solutions – this is Jez's ideal scenario. Encourage blue-sky thinking here and for him not to be shackled with practicalities. Encourage Jez to be creative and imaginative to generate energy. *Useful questions:* What do you ideally want instead?; What would be happening…? *and* What would you be doing/thinking/feeling?

2b Change Agenda – Help Jez to reflect upon his brainstorm ideas and formulate goals which are SMART (specific, measurable, achievable, realistic and timebound). *Useful questions:* What exactly is your goal with this?; Which of these feels best for you to address? *and* Which of this feels manageable to address?

2c Committment – Test this is the right goal for Jez to work on, and his commitment to it, before he moves into action. *Useful questions:* How will it be different for you when you do this…?; What are the benefits for you in doing this? *and* What are the disadvantages for you in doing this?

Stage 3: Finding a way forward

Aim of stage – To help the student with how to get to where they want.

Notes – Help Jez identify any strategies or actions to be able to move towards his identified goals as well as considering what/who could help or hinder this.

3a Possible actions – Help Jez to brainstorm strategies to achieve his goal. Again, encourage blue-sky thinking as ideas for action might come from wild ideas. *Useful questions:* What are the ways in which you could achieve…?; Who/what could help? *and* What has helped/hindered before?

3b Best fit strategies – Help Jez to focus from the brainstorm ideas on what is realistic for him and best fits with his circumstances and values. *Useful questions:* Which of these ideas appeals to you most?; Which of these ideas is most likely to work? *and* Which of these ideas do you have the resources to do?

3c Plan – Help Jez to plan the next steps by breaking down the goal into smaller steps for action. I must ensure this is Jez's plan and timescales, and not my own. *Useful questions:* What will you do first of all?; When will you achieve this by? *and* What will you need to do next?

End actions – Jez should have an action plan and begin to start working to this, whilst we still have regular meetings regarding the plan's progress. The plan/goal may need revising or adjusting.

Figure 7.1 Kate's preparation notes for meeting with Jez

Activity 7.3 Critical thinking

Read through Scenario 7.2, Kate's preparation notes for meeting with Jez.

1. What sort of communication style is Kate planning to use? How do we know this?
2. Think about your own communication style and skills. What are your strengths and weaknesses regarding communication skills? You might find this helpful to note down.

There is a model answer for this activity at the end of this chapter.

Egan's Skilled Helper model is useful to provide us with a framework or map to then be able to explore issues affecting the student, and help them to move to action. The model is designed to keep the student's agenda central, and we can see from Kate's plan in Scenario 7.2 and your critical thinking from Activity 7.3 that her role is to prompt and ask open-ended questions of Jez. She aims to enable him to end up with a plan of action for himself, developed from his own goals. Principles of good active listening are required throughout this interaction, and it's important that Kate doesn't try and add her own *solutions* but instead work in a very facilitative way to help Jez through the stages to reach his own. Not every student will need to address all three stages, and at times individuals may move back into previously addressed stages. Kate might find she uses her plan sequentially as she has written it, but she will also have to be prepared to work with Jez in all or any of the stages, and move backwards and forwards, as needed. It is not uncommon for the student to revisit earlier stages as the issue they first identified isn't the one they want most to address. Not all the stages will take an equal amount of time to work through, and this will vary depending on the student and also on their particular *issue*. Kate might find that it takes up all of one or maybe more meetings for Jez to work through stage 1, yet the following stages might then happen relatively quickly as the student begins to pick up pace as they move to action. The key with using this model is flexibility.

Supporting the failing student

Most students will achieve their required proficiencies in practice. Indeed, most students *in difficulty* who are provided with support, will go on to achieve and pass the placement. However, there are a few students whose performance is not able to meet the required standards even with extra support, and these students will need to be supported to fail practice. It is not always straightforward to be able to fail a student. *Failure to fail* is the term used when students who do not display satisfactory clinical performance are given a *pass* mark. Duffy's (2003) seminal work on *failing to fail* showed that mentors were sometimes passing students they thought should have failed. The reasons for this were that mentors lacked confidence in failing students and wanted to give students the *benefit of the doubt*. Failing to fail can have significant implications for the students and practice assessors involved, as well as an effect on nursing professionalism and in particular patient safety. Duffy's work led to a revision in the NMC (2008) guidance for those supporting practice assessments. However, more recent research has shown that failing to fail still occurs. Registrants involved in assessment decisions often struggle to deal with personality clashes, emotional blackmail, poor hygiene, aggression, punctuality and learning difficulties such as dyslexia (Lawson, 2010). Activity 7.4 offers you an opportunity to explore these issues further.

Activity 7.4   Leadership and management

Using any experiences you may have had in working with failing students, think about potential reasons why failing to fail still happens.

If you haven't had any direct experiences of working with failing students, you could ask your colleagues about their experiences. You might find it helpful to make a note of these.

There is a model answer at the end of this chapter that outlines common themes about failing to fail from the wider literature.

Assessment of competence is an essential component of the practice assessor's role. Activity 7.4 highlights that failing a student can be difficult for many reasons, and sometimes results in failing to fail.

Indicators of failing practice

Practice assessors are responsible for confirming students are capable and safe to practice. Chapter 6 details how we can assess competence of students during clinical practice. Earlier in this chapter, indicators of students being in difficulty were highlighted. However, there are also common indicators in a student's skills performance or behaviour, which could alert an assessor to the possibility of failure. Table 7.3 outlines common indicators of student practice failure from research undertaken by Duffy and Hardicre (2007a).

You might recognise some of the indicators from students you have already worked with and reflections from Activity 7.4.

Utilising the assessment process

One of the reasons Duffy (2003) found that contributed to registrants failing to fail was that those undertaking practice assessments lacked knowledge of the assessment

- Inconsistency in meeting the required level of competence for the stage of training;
- Inconsistent clinical performance;
- Lack of insight into weaknesses so unable to change following constructive feedback;
- Unsafe practice;
- Not responding appropriately to feedback;
- Lack of interest or motivation;
- Limited practical, interpersonal and communication skills;
- Absence of professional boundaries and/or poor professional behaviour;
- Experiencing continual poor health, feeling depressed, uncommitted, withdrawn, sad, tired or listless;
- Unreliability, persistent lateness/absence;
- Preoccupation with personal issues;
- Lack of theoretical knowledge.

Table 7.3   Common indicators of student practice failure (Duffy and Hardicre, 2007b)

process. As presented in Chapter 6, practice-based assessments should be conducted transparently, rigorously and fairly. It should be very clear for the student whether the assessment is formative or summative. Students should usually have at least three formal meetings with their practice assessor. There should be an initial assessment interview, mid-placement interview and final placement interview. These should occur for all students, and are particularly helpful for highlighting progression and any issues.

At the initial meeting, it is essential to discuss any learning needs and requirements. The student's documentation should be reviewed and then between assessor and student any learning objectives and action plans should be developed. Future meetings should be scheduled, and all this activity thoroughly documented.

The mid-placement interview is formative and it is crucial to highlight the student's progress towards their objectives and plans at this point. Any areas for development should be discussed here, especially if the practice assessor has any concerns about the student's progression. Any conversations of this nature along with any plans for development, records of extra support required and other actions, should be thoroughly documented. If there are concerns regarding progression at this point, it will also be necessary to contact the student's academic tutors who can provide additional support for the student as well as for the assessor. This could be their academic tutor or tutor who links from the AEI, and their contact details should be clearly outlined in the student's assessment book. This meeting is potentially the most critical in supporting failing students, due to its timing. It should provide an opportunity for any concerns to be addressed with the student, and support to be put in place to scaffold the rest of the placement. With additional support and action plans, the aim is for the student to be able to successfully progress and achieve their outcomes. Assessors should not leave the *failing* news to the last meeting where there is no chance of the student being able to correct the situation. Duffy (2003) found that mentors often failed to fail because of a fear that their decision would be *overruled* by the student's AEI. Students are only able to appeal a failed assessment decision if there are grounds on which to do so. If the assessor fails to highlight concerns at this mid-point, it would be a case for appeal as the student has not had time to address any weaknesses or flaws.

The final assessment interview will include summative assessment decisions and should take place towards the end of the placement. There should be no surprises for the student at this meeting, as concerns and progress have been discussed previously. The meeting is used to record a pass or fail grade for the placement. Each AEI will have its own set of documentation to use for these meetings and it is critical for the practice assessor to familiarise themselves with the documentation used in their area. It is also important for practice supervisors to be familiar with assessment documentation and how the student is progressing. Supervisors will be responsible for feeding into assessment decisions and will need to be cognisant of any objectives, action plans and additional support that have been planned. Activity 7.5 provides an opportunity for you to familiarise yourself with the assessment process in the documentation the students use in your specific workplace.

Activity 7.5   Leadership and management

Familiarise yourself with the assessment process included in the documentation of the students who access your practice area. Take note of who to contact should there be a cause for concern. Talk to experienced practice assessors in your practice area about their experiences of using the assessment process. You may wish to make some notes from this activity for your own development.

There is no correct answer to this activity as it relates to your own experiences.

Understanding the assessment process and the student's assessment requirements is essential for you to be able to make fair decisions about the student's competence and progression. If issues have arisen and extra support and opportunities have been provided, it might be the case that your student still fails to meet the standards and will fail the placement. Failing a student can be a difficult and unpleasant experience for the practice assessor, as well as the wider team involved in supporting the student. The important factor throughout this assessment process is that you seek support as early as possible for yourself as well as your student, if there are causes of concern regarding progression.

Student reactions to failing decisions

Upon hearing that they are underperforming or failing a placement, students can act in numerous ways. As with any bad news, it will take time to digest what is being said and you might find you need to repeat information given, or even write down information for the student. Table 7.4 outlines numerous student reactions to failing decisions. You might be familiar to these reactions if you have been involved in breaking bad news to patients or service users. It is likely you will already have transferable communication skills with delivering the bad news, in this instance to students instead of patients/service users.

Potential student reactions	Explanations for reactions
Denial, disbelief and shock	The student may have an inaccurate self-assessment of their own abilities and competence. Alternatively, they might have received differing feedback from other colleagues who gave them the *benefit of the doubt*.
Betrayal	The student might feel hurt that their practice assessor and/or supervisor who they felt they got along well with, could fail them.
Sadness and upset	The student might cry or be tearful.
Anger, aggression and denial	The student may shout or verbally abuse their practice assessor, accusing them of bias or victimisation.
Blaming others	The student might blame personality clashes or accuse the assessor of underperforming themselves. The student may blame others for giving them the wrong information. This could be the assessor, previous assessors, other members of the team, academics or even other students.
Bargaining, coercion	Some student nurses can use coercive and manipulative behaviour to try and gain a successful outcome to their practice learning assessment. They might try and bargain with the assessor to change their assessment decision. This often results in causing assessors to feel guilty.
Relief	Some students may be relieved and accept a failed assessment. This might be when they themselves have recognised some clinical weakness or areas that need additional work.

Table 7.4 Student reactions to failing decisions (adapted from Duffy and Hardicre, 2007a; Hunt et al., 2016)

An awareness of potential reactions to failing news can really help us prepare for those difficult conversations. These potential reactions also highlight the importance of ensuring you and the student are supported with this process. An academic from the student's programme will ideally be present when news of failing is first presented to the student and then at each meeting where progression is discussed.

Managing failing students

Any concerns about a student's performance should be raised as early as possible. The aim is to provide feedback that can *correct* the concern and support the student to pass. Feedback should be both written and verbal and you may need to arrange several opportunities to keep discussing this so that the student is very clear on what they need to do to improve. Feedback is essential and Chapter 5 outlines principles of good feedback that are particularly helpful here.

Documenting concerns in the student's assessment documentation makes these clear and transparent for the student and all those involved in supporting them. This is especially important if your student is being supervised in practice by a team of supervisors, providing continuity of approach and focus on a shared goal. Evidence should also be documented of related performance and behaviours that are causing the concern. Documenting particular examples can help the student (and others) to better understand assessment decisions. Documentation should be factual; non-judgmental; identify strengths and weaknesses and be specific. All related assessment conversations and details of any supportive measures in place should be recorded.

If issues have been identified, it is important to involve academics from the student's programme and also allocate more supervised time for the student from practice supervisors and assessors. When making an assessment decision, a practice assessor should judge if some minor issues can be accepted as part of the student's continued development, or whether issues are so serious and have not been resolved, and failure is inevitable.

Duffy and Hardicre (2007b) offer the following practical tips for dealing with managing failing students:

- Ensure all meetings take place in a private area where you will not be disturbed.
- Invite the student to undertake a self-assessment.
- Formulate an action plan.
- Clearly identify evidence of success or improvements.
- Formulate learning objectives for the next meeting.
- Identify appropriate learning opportunities to meet the objectives.
- Identify additional knowledge required and where the student can access this.
- Plan the date of the next meeting and have regular progress meetings.

Practice assessors and practice supervisors should remain positive and supportive when working with a failing student. Students will have an opportunity to develop over the wider programme even if they have not met the final standard required to pass the particular placement you are assessing. If they have failed the placement, the academic course team will decide on next options for the student. This might be re-taking a particular placement or set of practice assessments, or could be moving to an earlier progression point of the course. In some cases, students will be required to leave the course. These decisions are made following a thorough review of the student's profile and any particular assessment patterns. All those involved in supporting assessment decisions should have a sound understanding of the assessment process and be confident in failing a student should they need to. Most importantly as practice assessors and supervisors, you must be confident that patients and service users will be in safe hands if the student continues to proceed beyond the placement.

Chapter summary

After reading this chapter and completing the activities, we can better recognise and support a student who is in difficulty or failing their summative practice assessment. Although stress is an everyday part of life, prolonged stress can be unhelpful and can lead to undesirable behaviours. Nurses and midwives at any level of experience can exhibit undesirable behaviours when in a stressed state. Being a student with the pressures of assessment often adds another layer of stress for an individual.

The issues causing students to be in difficulty or to fail are often complex and multi-faceted. Through supportive practice assessment and practice supervision we can work with students to help them address issues. Egan's Skilled Helper model can be useful when supporting students in difficulty as this model puts the student firmly at the centre of any activity. The model's particular strength is the structure it provides, especially as we establish and embed our developing skills. Utilising the assessment process to manage failing students can provide us with a framework to ensure our decisions are fair, transparent and based on evidence. We must be confident that the assessment decisions we are involved with have patient and service user safety at their core.

Activity answers

Activity 7.1: Critical thinking (p127)

There is no correct answer to this activity if it relates to your own experiences. If you have considered Jez's stress signs, symptoms and behaviours from Scenario 7.1, you may have noted the following:

Emotional symptoms	Mental symptoms	Changes from normal behaviour
• Negative or depressive feeling • Disappointment with yourself • Loss of motivation, commitment and confidence *(Jez says negative comments about his abilities.* *Uses terms:* totally messed up, it's all gone downhill *and* I just can't seem to get anything right. *He seems to lack confidence and motivation to work with the patient again)*	• Lack of clarity • Lack of ability to prioritise *(Jez isn't able to clearly assess what he is required to do as he leaves the busy ward. He isn't able to prioritise direct patient care; instead he is investigating information about treatment procedures.)*	• Changes in attendance such as avoidance. *(Jez has taken himself away from the situation he is finding difficult. In this case, direct patient care, and gone to do something different. He seems reluctant to be directly involved in care again with this patient.)*

Activity 7.3: Critical thinking (p134)

1. You will have noticed that Kate plans to use active listening skills in this meeting. This means she will make a conscious effort to hear the words that Jez is saying along with the complete message he is communicating. This involves using open-ended questions, reflection and summarising skills to be absolutely clear of the student's message.

2. There is no model answer for this question as it involves your own experience. However, studies have found that many health professionals don't routinely use active listening skills (Arnold and Boggs, 2015). Instead, we are used to using a series of closed-ended questions and making quick judgements to then offer our advice. Good communication skills require a high level of self-awareness so understanding our own style and any development needs is important. If you would like to read further about active listening skills, check out the online resource provided by NHS Improvement (no date) at https://improvement.nhs.uk/documents/2085/active-listening.pdf.

Activity 7.4: Leadership and management (p135)

There is no correct answer to this activity if it relates to your own experiences. However, Hughes et al. (2016) undertook a systematic integrative literature review to determine what is currently known about the issue of *failure to fail* in undergraduate nursing and midwifery programmes. From this research, five main themes emerged why failing to fail still happens. Your list may contain similar issues to those noted by the researchers. These themes were:

1. Failing a student is difficult to do.

2. Failing a student is an emotional experience for all parties involved.

3. Confidence and skills to fail are required to fail students.

4.   AEI support is required to fail students.

5.   Some student characteristics make failing even more difficult.

The researchers concluded that *failure to fail* is still a real issue that has many complex facets.

Further reading and useful websites

Egan's Skilled Helper model, developed by gp-training.net. Available at: **www.gp-training.net/ training/communication_skills/mentoring/egan.htm**. This online resource was developed to support General Practitioners and provides some further detail on applying the model to support students in difficulty.

Hughes, LJ, Mitchell, M and Johnston, AN (2016) 'Failure to fail' in nursing: a catch phrase or a real issue? A systematic integrative literature review. *Nurse Education in Practice*, 20: 54–63. This article details the issues involved in failing a student and the emotional processes involved for both assessors and students. It also highlights the implications of failure to fail for the profession, organisations and patient safety.

Chapter 8 Developing yourself as a supervisor and/or assessor

Standards Framework for Nursing and Midwifery Education. Part 1 of Realising Professionalism: Standards for Education and Training (NMC, 2018d)

This chapter will address the standards in heading **3: Student empowerment**.

3.2 Students are empowered and supported to become resilient, caring, reflective and life-long learners who are capable of working in inter-professional and inter-agency teams.

and **4: Educators and assessors**.

4.1 Theory and practice learning and assessment are facilitated effectively and objectively by appropriately qualified and experienced professionals with necessary expertise for their educational roles.

The Code: Professional Standards of Practice and Behaviour for Nurses and Midwives (NMC, 2015)

This chapter most closely aligns with the following professional standards.

Prioritise people

1.1 treat people with kindness, respect and compassion.

Practise effectively

6.2 maintain the knowledge and skills you need for safe and effective practice.

7.1 use terms that people in your care, colleagues and the public can understand.

8.2 maintain effective communication with colleagues.

8.4 work with colleagues to evaluate the quality of your work and that of the team.

9.1 provide honest, accurate and constructive feedback to colleagues.

9.2 gather and reflect on feedback from a variety of sources, using it to improve your practice and performance.

(Continued)

(Continued)

9.3 deal with differences of professional opinion with colleagues by discussion and informed debate, respecting their views and opinions and behaving in a professional way at all times.

9.4 support students' and colleagues' learning to help them develop their professional competence and confidence.

Preserve safety

16.6 protect anyone you have management responsibility for from any harm, detriment, victimisation or unwarranted treatment after a concern is raised.

Promote professionalism and trust

20.8 act as a role model of professional behaviour for students and newly qualified nurses and midwives to aspire to.

22.3 keep your knowledge and skills up to date, taking part in appropriate and regular learning and professional development activities that aim to maintain and develop your competence and improve your performance.

Chapter aims

After reading this chapter, you will be able to:

- define and describe mental wellbeing and resilience and understand their value within the context of supporting learners;
- describe models and techniques to develop resilience and mental wellbeing;
- consider the usefulness of resilience and mental wellbeing should things *go wrong*;
- assess and plan for your continuing professional development needs;
- apply your knowledge and skills to develop your colleagues and profession.

Introduction

The evidence indicates that being resilient is a protective factor for healthcare professionals (Dean, 2012). Much has been written about the value of resilience in promoting mental wellbeing and protecting healthcare practitioners from fatigue, burnout and ill-health (Koen et al., 2011). Resilience and mental wellbeing can have a positive effect on absenteeism and is therefore of importance to the NHS where costs due to ill-health were £1 billion in the three-year period preceding 2013 (Anonymous,

2013). However, although much has been written about resilience in this context, little is known about the impact of resilience in the context of supporting learners and this chapter will focus on what we do know. It will also consider how resilience can protect patients from harm through enabling professionals to stay well; can support students who escalate concerns; and can help registrants fail students who do not meet the required levels of competence. The chapter will then move on to look at your how your skills as a supervisor can be used to support your own and your colleagues' professional development, thereby developing your profession as a whole.

What is resilience?

The importance of resilience when experiencing significant life events such as war and disasters has been understood for some time. However, resilience has more recently been studied in the area of health and healthcare. There is evidence to indicate that being a resilient healthcare practitioner can not only support our physical and emotional wellbeing but can offer a level of *protection* in stressful situations, or *when things go wrong* (Seymour-Walsh, 2016).

What do we mean by resilience? The literature suggests that resilient individuals, even after experiencing an adverse event, can function at their previous levels. Some may also experience increases in autonomy and changes in their perspective on life. In other words, these individuals can change adversity into a positive life experience and *bounce back* stronger than before. Although there are many definitions of resilience, there are a number of shared features. These are:

- the ability to bounce back;
- the ability to hold on to hope and optimism;
- the belief that you have some influence or control over a situation;
- a sense of self-compassion and knowing not to blame oneself;
- the knowledge that resilience is protective.

Resilience can help healthcare practitioners cope with the stresses of the constant decision-making and risk management that they face. Resilient practice supervisors/assessors are strong role models to learners and help them develop their own resilience. It is a powerful tool to develop and have in both your practitioner and supervisor/assessor tool box! Increasing our own self-awareness about our resilience helps us to identify areas that we may find particularly difficult. Activity 8.1 will help you to develop your self-awareness of your resilience.

Now that you have completed the checklist in Activity 8.1, think about someone you believe to be resilient. This may be someone you have worked with, or still do, or possibly someone you know who has dealt with a difficult situation or life event. Think about their characteristics and attributes and how these link to them being a resilient individual Now go back to the definitions and descriptions of resilience and identify

Activity 8.1   Reflection

Resilience checklist

In the table list what helps you feel resilient and what erodes your resilience.

Helps	Erodes
e.g. The support I get from my work colleagues	*e.g. Working without a regular lunch break*

There is no model answer as this activity is based upon your own reflection.

any *gaps* you have and consider how you might go about acquiring these skills. You may yourself have a coach, supervisor or someone you trust with whom you could talk this over. Consider this as part of your resilience journey and invest in it as it will help protect you for the rest of your career.

Scenario 8.1

This scenario outlines a day in the life of Tina, an experienced community mental health nurse and practice supervisor, who is working with Daphne, a third-year student nurse.

Tina and Daphne are chatting in Tina's car on their way to a visit. Daphne tells Tina that she is struggling with working in the community and not enjoying this placement. She said that she finds it difficult not having a range of colleagues immediately accessible to her. Also, she misses the familiarity of the ward environment, and the sense of 'control' she has there.

Today, they have been out together to see John. John has paranoid schizophrenia and is feeling very suspicious of Daphne and wonders if she is really a spy. Tina herself is also finding the situation with John hard. She has known him a long time and finds it difficult when he is struggling. However, Tina feels she is able to keep on top of her emotions. Daphne fed back to her that she sees Tina as a positive role model as she remains very caring and compassionate with John while explaining how potentially serious the situation is. Daphne told Tina she hoped she could be as kind and truthful in similar situations.

> *When they get back to the office, Tina and Daphne hand over to their colleagues and Tina discloses how sad she feels about John's situation and that he may have to be admitted to the hospital: something he really hates.*
>
> *Later that day, Tina tells Daphne that she is looking forward to a long swim after work because it helps her relax. Also, she has clinical supervision booked in for tomorrow and this is something she prioritises. The situation with John will be top of her list to discuss. Next week she has a meeting of a journal club she is member of to discuss developments in her professional field. She enjoys this time learning with and supporting her colleagues. Tina asks Daphne what she plans to do in order to unwind. Daphne doesn't know.*

As highlighted in Scenario 8.1, care and compassion are seen as important aspects of resilience. The *6Cs* were launched in 2012 as part of the document *Compassion in Practice* (Cummings and Bennett, 2012) and encompassed the following attributes: care, compassion, courage, commitment, communication and competence. Although the key driver was about adopting and conveying these attributes with patients and carers they are highly transferable to supporting learners in practice. The summary in Figure 8.1 provides an overview of Duffy's (2015) article: Integrating the 6Cs of nursing into mentorship practice.

Complete Activity 8.2 immediately after reading this and consider how adopting the 6Cs in your practice may help you and your learners become more resilient.

Duffy (2015) highlights the importance of role modelling and how both good and bad behaviours and attitudes have a powerful impact on learners.

Care – This can be developed by conveying a sense of belonging to the learners, showing that they are welcome and are part of the team. Encouraging early and active engagement in caring for patients also helps.

Compassion – This can be developed through acknowledging the emotional labour of the work we do and encouraging reflection and including learners in any debriefing following traumatic events. Thinking aloud and sharing your thoughts including how the situation may be impacting on a patient and their family demonstrates empathy and compassionate practice to the learner.

Competence – Being supportive in your role as supervisor/assessor enables learners to more readily achieve competence and there are a number of techniques you can use to help develop their psychomotor skills and thereby acquire competence. Supervisor/assessors need to confidently engage learners in a discussion around the evidence base to support their practice and care delivery and the decision around competence.

(Continued)

(Continued)

Communication – Learners need to be given opportunities to develop their communication skills. Before meeting with a patient explain to the learner the purpose of the meeting and what you hope to achieve. This will help the learner make sense of the conversation and develop their communication skills. Just as important is role-modelling effective communication with members of the wider team, including the university.

Courage – Demonstrate to learners you have the passion and courage to innovate and transform practice; to question received wisdom and practices and to speak out if care isn't good enough. It also takes courage as an assessor to take the decision to fail a learner if they are not achieving the competencies.

Commitment – Demonstrate commitment to the supervisor/assessor role and the learner through preparing yourself with the placement documentation, the course and the competencies they need to achieve. This goes beyond the individual and should span the learning environment and the whole team where everyone is committed to creating a positive learning environment for learners.

Figure 8.1   Overview of integrating the 6Cs of nursing into practice learning

As you will have noticed from reading the summary in Figure 8.1, role-modelling is an important aspect of supervising learners.

Activity 8.2   Leadership and management

Identify one change you wish to make against each of the 6Cs in relation to your own practice. You might wish to make a copy of this for your portfolio and discuss at your appraisal.

There is no model answer for this activity as it is based upon your own reflections.

Acting upon the changes identified in Activity 8.2 will help us to become more resilient. Practice supervisors/assessors who demonstrate the 6Cs also role-model the behaviours of resilient individuals. This can help their learners to become more resilient and will help them throughout their career. In Scenario 8.1, Daphne has already noticed that Tina is *very caring and compassionate with John* and is therefore successfully role-modelling these behaviours. Daphne may wish to focus on developing in these areas herself.

Mental wellbeing and resilience

Mental wellbeing is when a person is able to develop their potential and work productively and creatively. This enables us to build strong and positive relationships with others and contribute to our community. There are two key aspects of mental wellbeing: feeling good and functioning well. Although it is important to feel happy and engaged, of equal importance is our sense of purpose in the world and what we can add to it. Many people who choose nursing or midwifery as a career have strong vocational drive to help others and this latter aspect of mental wellbeing may be even stronger for them. McDermid et al.'s (2016) study of new nurse academics identified three factors that helped them transition into their new role. These are:

- having a mentor and developing supportive work relationships;
- focusing on positive feedback and experiences;
- reflecting on difficult situations and developing as a result of this.

This learning can be applied to students as well as ourselves as they too transition into new roles. In 2008 the UK government commissioned a mental capital and wellbeing project (Kirkwood et al., 2014); details of this can be found in Activity 8.4. The project identified factors that promote mental wellbeing. The *five ways to wellbeing* were identified as:

- connect – feeling close to and valued by others;
- be active – enjoying regular physical activity;
- take notice – being mindful and taking time to notice things around you;
- learn – engaging with new learning;
- give – getting involved in community events.

Activity 8.3   Evidence-based practice and research

1. Visit Mind's website, which includes more information on the five ways to wellbeing. (Available at: **www.mind.org.uk/workplace/mental-health-at-work/taking-care-of-yourself/five-ways-to-wellbeing/**)

2. Consider each one and identify something you already do or commit to doing something new. Try to ensure you have something against each domain.

3. Next go back to the scenario and identify any activities mentioned that fit against any of the *five ways*.

There is a model answer to the second part of the activity at the end of the chapter.

Models to help develop your learners' resilience

Activity 8.3 highlighted some basic activities for wellbeing but there are a number of models that can help develop wellbeing and resilience. Aspects of these models can be used as part of your day-to-day practice when supporting learners. We will now apply Egan's (2013) Skilled Helper model and the cognitive behavioural approach. However, regardless of which model you use they all have the following elements:

- they have boundaries and ground rules – you are the practice supervisor/assessor not the best friend, nor are you their parent;
- they value the *core conditions* namely genuineness, warmth and empathy;
- they promote listening and communication skills, including reflecting and paraphrasing;
- they are learner focused – although you have specific tasks to complete try to keep the learning focused on their needs. As you know, every learner is different and will have a different set of experiences; strengths; deficits and concerns.

Egan's (2013) Skilled Helper model is discussed here (as well as in Chapter 7) because it is concise and can be applied to supporting learners in practice. Let's consider how we can apply the three stages of Egan's model to a common scenario: a student's first couple of weeks on a new placement (Table 8.1).

Stage	Attributes, behaviours and activities
Stage 1: telling the story	Spend the first few days working with the learner to understand what they feel are their strengths and areas for development. Ask about the situations in which they feel more and less comfortable; the tasks and skills they are competent in and those they need to develop. Elicit what they have learnt from previous placement experiences. Encourage the learner to *take control* of the discussion and try to avoid jumping in with answers and advice. Communication skills such as *conveying empathy and compassion will help in this first stage.*
Stage 2: the preferred picture	Once the relationship has been established you can start to find out from the learner what they see as their goals. How are they feeling about the placement? Is it an area they are familiar with or is it new to them? What do they absolutely need to achieve and are there some further, more individualised goals? Is there anything they feel they need to *conquer,* for example the dreaded injection or ward round! This is also the time for you to be explicit and honest about what your requirements are and any early observations and feedback. *Attributes and skills such as courage and communication will help with this stage.*
Stage 3: finding a way forward	Once you are both clear about what needs to be achieved you can start to create a plan to enable the learner to get there. They can construct this and you can adapt it together. This may include the need to spend time with other practitioners, or more personally presenting information to the full multi-disciplinary team. *Skills and attributes such as competence and commitment are important here.*

Table 8.1 Applying the Skilled Helper model

The cognitive behavioural approach suggests that how we react to events is largely determined by our views of them, not by the events themselves. Therefore, how we think about a situation influences how we feel about it and subsequently how we behave. Through examining and re-evaluating some of our less helpful thoughts and being more self-compassionate we can develop and try out alternative viewpoints and behaviours that may be more effective in problem-solving and developing resilience (Kemper et al., 2015). The ABC model (Powell, 2009) helps to further explain this:

A is the **antecedent, or activating event**. This is usually something that happened to the person or something they witnessed

B is their **behaviour** and

C the **consequence** of their behaviour.

Scenario 8.2

This scenario focuses on David who is a new practice supervisor. He is supporting Ali, a second-year nurse. They are working on a busy surgical unit.

Ali and David attended the ward handover where Ali handed over a patient called Mr Adeboah. Ali forgot to inform the team that Mr Adeboah was nil by mouth in preparation for a procedure later. Later on, Mr Adeboah was offered a cup of tea, which he accepted, and then his procedure had to be cancelled. The anaesthetist and surgeon complained to the ward manager. David feels very embarrassed that he didn't notice Ali's error and he knows he is accountable. He thinks people are now questioning his competence. He's also worried about the impact this has had on patient care and wonders if this could be considered a near miss. Now when he supervises students he is constantly double/triple checking they have passed on all the information, and does not allow them to hand over patient care anymore. This is affecting his students' ability to develop their skills.

Now that you have familiarised yourself with the scenario, it's time to complete Activity 8.4 and try to apply the ABC model to it.

We can see from Scenario 8.2 and Activity 8.4 what David thinks about the situation (*I'm an embarrassment, people will think I am incompetent*) influences how he feels (embarrassed/shame) and how he behaves (restricting students' autonomy and double-checking everything). The relationship between these three elements of the ABC model is the key hypothesis in the cognitive behavioural approach (Neenan and Dryden, 2013). This negative spiral may have an impact on David's resilience and ability to *bounce back* as well as role-modelling negative resilience behaviours to his students.

Activity 8.4   Critical thinking

Read Scenario 8.2 and identify the following:

A the antecedent or activating event

B the beliefs

C the consequence

There is a model answer at the end of the chapter.

However, challenging or disputing the negative thoughts can transform how we think and what we do. The addition of D (dispute) to the model prompts an individual to challenge their negative beliefs. For example different thoughts for David such as *I should have checked with Ali that he handed that information over but I didn't I was so busy it dropped off my list. That doesn't mean I'm incompetent; everyone, even the best supervisors make mistakes.*

This may lead to him acting differently, which is the E (or new event) to the model. An example of this might involve David observing Ali at the next handover and checking his competence around verbal communication. This will lead to a change in David's behaviour where he will no longer double/triple-check everything, however minor, and alter a change in his emotional state where he feels less apprehensive and embarrassed.

Adopting a seven-step problem-solving sequence (Wasik, 1984, cited in Palmer, 2008) can help practice supervisors or assessors to develop skills to challenge thinking and change behaviours. In Table 8.2 this is applied to David's situation from Scenario 8.2.

Steps	Questions and actions	David's thoughts and actions
Problem identification	What is the concern?	I've lost confidence in myself as a supervisor.
Goal selection	What do I want?	To feel more confident and allow students some autonomy.
Generation of alternatives	What can I do?	Gradually allow students more autonomy once they have demonstrated competence.

Consideration of consequences	What might happen?	A student might still make a mistake: there's always that risk!
Target	What is the most feasible solution?	Start with patient handover.
Implementation	Now do it!	Starting tomorrow I will gradually allow more autonomy.
		I'll also talk to Ash, he's an experienced supervisor and assessor and someone I trust.
Evaluation	Did it work?	I'll evaluate in one month and get feedback from a range of colleagues, patients and learners.

Table 8.2   A seven-step approach to problem solving

Dealing with difficult situations

As healthcare professionals we are constantly dealing with complexity and stressful events and resilience can help us remain buoyant in the face of these. The pace of change in the NHS is fast and constant and this in itself requires us to be resilient. The NMC has highlighted the importance of resilience to the profession in numerous documents and the role it has in enabling registrants to continue to deliver high-quality care. However, we are sometimes faced with very difficult situations or times when things *go wrong*. It is these situations when we need our resilience more than ever in order to bounce back and, if possible, learn from them. In the context of supporting learners this might be when we make the decision to fail a student or if a student we are supporting has escalated their concerns about patient safety or sub-standard care.

Duffy (2003) identified the phenomenon of *failing to fail*, which indicated mentors were passing students they thought should have failed. Research carried out by Jervis and Tilki (2011) indicates that this phenomenon is still evident but also found that when mentors do make the decision to fail a student it places intense pressure on them. This is covered in more detail in Chapter 7. Mentors who made the decision to fail a student expressed a range of concerns including fear of being subjected to a grievance by the student; worrying that their competence as a mentor might be questioned; having the decision overturned by the university; feeling emotionally blackmailed by the student through to experiencing stress and sleepless nights. There are a number of recommendations to help supervisor/assessors/mentors to make the right decisions and support them through this. These include assessor preparation programmes that build in opportunities to reflect on and critically analyse experiences in a safe and supportive environment. Also, forums to help supervisors and assessors manage difficult situations arising from referring students in practice assessments (Jervis and Tilki, 2010). The previous chapters have explored the benefits of a team approach to supporting learners. Also, the creation of the distinct roles of supervisor and assessor promotes objectivity and separation between supervision and assessment. This may mean there is less emotional toil placed on assessors who fail students.

All learners, whether registrants or students, have a duty to escalate concerns about any poor or dangerous patient care they witness. If students do this during placement, you will need to support them with this. The stress people experience as a result of *whistleblowing* is well documented and a compassionate, supportive response can help the student deal with this (McDonald and Ahern, 2002). Students should be informed at the start of any placement how they can raise concerns and it is recommended they raise any concerns with you initially and also with the AEI. The NMC Code (NMC, 2015) has many standards relating to raising concerns about public safety. AEIs that deliver pre-registration nurse and midwife education programmes have a protocol readily available to students to assist them to raise any concerns. These protocols should be prominent in clinical areas as this sends a clear message to students that the practice area is open, transparent and takes any concerns seriously. It is during these very difficult situations that we need to protect and promote our mental wellbeing, although it is often easy to overlook this. Practising these techniques when things are going relatively smoothly will set up good habits for when we need to rely on them the most.

Assessing and planning for your continuing professional development

Now that you are developing your role as a supervisor and/or assessor, the next step is to think about your continuing professional development needs in relation to supporting learners.

Continuing professional development or CPD has a number of definitions but it is the process by which registrants engage in, record and reflect on a range of learning activities and experiences to enhance practice and maintain competence. CPD is a professional requirement for nurses and midwives. Our regulator, the NMC, requires all registrants to engage in CPD and return evidence of this as part of the revalidation process (NMC, 2017a). Although there are no legal requirements for employers to support registrants' CPD, many do. This is usually financially and/or through protected study time as CPD is a critical tool in delivering improved patient health outcomes; ensuring a high-quality health workforce and supporting staff to be safer, more effective and happier (RCN, 2016a).

CPD can take various forms and includes activities such as formal modules and courses that attract academic credit; conference attendance; working with particular colleagues or attendance at work-based learning events. Learning can be face-to-face or online. It also includes keeping up to date with contemporary issues through reading journal articles and books. We may learn with experts in the field including service users, carers and researchers. Many nurses have formal conversations about their CPD needs at their annual appraisal and as part of the NMC revalidation process (2017a). You should prepare for these meetings by considering what you believe are your strengths and which areas you would like to develop and then construct an action plan to help you get there – highlighting any support you might need. Consider short-term, medium-term and long-term goals. Ask at your place of work if there is a buddying or coaching scheme: someone to talk this through with. Professional body websites have invaluable resources and toolkits around career planning and professional development and you may wish to spend time accessing these.

You may find it useful to review your CPD needs against the *four pillars of advanced practice* (Health Education England, 2017). These are the four areas that professionals who are working at an advanced level should be competent in: clinical practice; leadership and management; education and research. What do you need to do to enhance your competence in these areas? You may decide you wish to focus on one area in particular. For instance, you may be interested in a career in nursing or midwifery education either in practice or at a AEI. If that's the case, you could look at job descriptions for such roles and identify the areas you need to develop. Also, get in touch with your local AEI and ask about opportunities such as guest lecturing in your areas of expertise, secondments and courses that can support your professional career development. Employers may fund or part-fund a course or you may be eligible for a grant from professional organisations such as the RCN. Although it may not be an immediate goal, you can still begin to develop your skill set and experience now.

Developing and supporting colleagues and the profession

As a practice supervisor and/or assessor you are a role model to others, demonstrating practice enhancement by actively engaging in CPD, and importantly changing practice as a result of this. This conveys a strong message to students and colleagues. You can achieve this by extending your role beyond supporting students. In addition, you can support your colleagues in developing and thereby developing the profession. Some *easy wins* in achieving this are:

- acting as a mentor, coach, preceptor or *buddy* to new or junior staff;
- delivering a learning event to colleagues on supporting students;
- co-ordinating activities to support the best use of evidence in practice such as a journal club;
- facilitating forums or communities of practice for other supervisors/assessors;
- undertaking appraisals with staff you manage;
- engaging in a reflective discussion (part of the NMC revalidation process);
- acting as a confirmer (part of the NMC revalidation process).

These examples provide an opportunity to support colleagues with their professional and career development goals and for you to provide feedback. However, you can encourage colleagues to step out of their *comfort zones* and consider other activities as part of their CPD. These could include shadowing leaders within the organisation, membership of strategic or clinical excellence groups, presentations at conferences or getting involved in a service improvement project. The range of CPD opportunities is almost limitless as you will find when undertaking Activity 8.5. Colleagues should be encouraged to think more widely and be creative! Having a nursing presence in service improvement projects for instance can have an impact on service design and delivery and ultimately patient care.

Activity 8.5 Leadership and management

Make some time to sit down with a colleague and discuss their CPD goals. This may be someone who is new to your area or someone you are buddying. Use Egan's model to understand what is important to them and define their goals. Capture the actions and make time to meet up to review them. After the meeting reflect on your involvement and include this in your own portfolio. Consider what went well, what you could have done differently and what you might change for your next meeting as a result of this learning.

There is no model answer as this activity is based upon your own experience.

Hopefully, you will find that Activity 8.5 helps colleagues to formalise their CPD goals. This can directly link professional development activities and the impact on patient outcomes. It can be a particularly powerful way to motivate individuals including those who lack confidence or are new to a clinical area.

Chapter summary

As a result of reading this chapter and completing the activities you should clearly see the importance of resilience and mental wellbeing to the placement learning context and your developing role. Your skills as a supervisor and/or assessor can be developed by applying knowledge and strategies from everyday techniques (five ways to wellbeing) and from more formal models (Egan and cognitive behavioural approaches). This chapter has highlighted that looking after our mental wellbeing can enhance our resilience and help us cope with the stresses associated with being a health professional. They can be particularly useful in enabling us to *bounce back* from very difficult situations. The importance of CPD in improving service delivery and care is highlighted, not only your own CPD but also through supporting others to engage in this activity.

Activity answers

Activity 8.3: Evidence-based practice and research (p149)

In relation to the scenario, the activities that fit against the *five ways* are:

- connect – Tina talked with her colleagues;
- be active – Tina was going swimming;
- take notice – Daphne noticed how caring and compassionate Tina was;
- learn – Tina engaged in clinical supervision;
- give – Tina is a member of a journal club.

Activity 8.4: Critical thinking (p152)

	Applying the ABC to the scenario	Recap
A = Activating event	In the scenario this is the anaesthetist and surgeon complaining to the ward manager.	This can be something that we directly experience, as in David's case or something we observe, e.g. a car crash.
B = Beliefs	he is worried that the error could be considered a *near miss* … He thinks people are now questioning his competence. He thinks he is an embarrassment to his profession.	Beliefs can also be termed thoughts or cognitions. The cognitive behavioural approach is based on evidence that negative beliefs or thoughts give rise to unpleasant physical feelings and affect our mood and behaviours.
C = Consequence first one is behaviour	David is constantly double/triple checking that students have passed on all the information and does not allow them to *hand over* patient care anymore (behaviours – what he has started and stopped doing).	There are three aspects to consequence. Behaviours are usually observable to others. However, they may not be. For example someone might count in threes when they think of a stressful situation. This can't be observed by others but it is an intentional act.
C = Consequence second one is feelings (physical)	He has butterflies in his stomach when he thinks about a student engaging in pre-operative care.	Physical sensations can be very unpleasant, and people may think they are about to faint etc. The behaviours someone adopts may be a way of reducing the physical sensation, e.g. avoiding a situation which is stressful.

(Continued)

(Continued)

	Applying the ABC to the scenario	Recap
C = Consequence second one is feelings (emotional)	He has been feeling apprehensive about students asking about being involved in pre-operative procedures (feelings emotional). He feels embarrassed.	Emotions such as apprehension, anxiety and depression are commonly reported.

Further reading

Egan, G (2013) *The Skilled Helper: A Problem-management and Opportunity-development Approach to Helping.* Belmont, CA: Cengage Learning – A great book if you want to find out more about this mentoring/helping model.

Powell, T (2009) *The Mental Health Handbook 3rd edition: A Cognitive Behavioural Approach.* London: Speechmark Publishing Ltd. This is really is a handbook. Describes the cognitive behavioural approach and has some excellent handouts and activities.

Useful websites

Health Education England – pages on Advanced Clinical Practice, which includes information on the four pillars you may wish to assess your CPD needs against.

NMC – pages with information on revalidation and the revalidation process. It includes a range of templates you can complete to provide evidence to support your revalidation.

Glossary

Approved Education Institution (AEI)   this is an educational institution, usually a university, that has been approved by the NMC to deliver NMC-approved programmes. In addition to the institution being approved, individual courses must also be approved (see **NMC-approved programme**).

autonomy   in relation to nursing practice is linked to the ability to demonstrate competence by working independently and confidently making decisions, exercising clinical reasoning and judgement.

Care Quality Commission (CQC)   is the independent regulator of health and adult social care in England. It has a number of standards that all health and social care services must meet. It regulates a wide range of services including hospitals, GP practices, dental practices, ambulance services, care homes and home-care agencies. The CQC monitors and inspect services to see whether they are safe, effective, caring, responsive and well led.

communities of practice (CoP)   a community of practice is a group of individuals who come together (face-to-face or online) to generate and share ideas and seek solutions to common problems. They may not regularly work together, but will be experiencing similar problems. CoPs are more effective when they are supported by organisations and employers while being allowed to create and innovate. They can be used in education to focus on areas such as assessment methods or ways to enhance distance learning. In practice, they may be used to innovate around options to hospital admission.

empowerment   is when individuals are given opportunities to work on issues that are important to them. They are seen as part of the solution and are encouraged to take control and make decisions.

experiential learning   is learning from experience. It has a structured approach thst includes reflecting on and making sense of our experiences in order to make any necessary changes to improve our practice.

fitness to practise (FtP)   is a term used by the NMC. Being fit to practise requires a nurse or midwife to have the skills, knowledge, good health and good character to do their job safely and effectively. All registered nurses and midwives must follow the NMC Code. If an allegation is made to the NMC regarding a nurse or midwife's fitness to practise it will investigate whether the registrant meets its standards for skills, education and behaviour. As a result, the NMC may remove an individual from the register permanently or for a set period of time.

formative assessment is a type of assessment that can be used throughout a period of study. It gives individuals the opportunity to see how they are progressing and provide feedback on their performance to enable them to improve.

interprofessional learning a range of professionals learning *with, from and about* each other. There are shared learning opportunities including modules and practice learning.

mentoring and coaching are often used interchangeably. Coaching is usually a short-term relationship focusing on specific goals or development area. The coach may have expertise in an area the person wishes to develop. Mentoring is a longer-term relationship and has a less focused approach. It may be concerned with longer-tem development and career planning.

multi-professional working more than one professional group working in an area such as a ward or community setting. There may be some sharing of tasks and responsibilities.

NMC-approved programme this is a course that has been approved by the NMC as meeting its standards and requirements. NMC-approved programmes enable people who have successfully completed them to be added to the NMC register or have their qualifications recorded on the NMC register. For example, a pre-registration nursing programme that, on successful completion, entitles someone to register as a nurse with the NMC.

NMC revalidation this was introduced by the NMC in April 2016 to replace PREP (post-registration education and practice). It is a process that occurs every three years and all NMC registrants must follow it to maintain their registration with the NMC.

Observed Structured Clinical Examination (OSCE) is an assessment of clinical competence carried out in a structured and objective way. It is commonly used in pre-registration and postgraduate programmes. The OSCE format often comprises a number of assessment *stations* that students rotate around with various tasks to complete to assess competence. Stations may include history taking or using a clinical screening tool.

pedagogy is concerned with the theory and practice of teaching. It is interested in how we learn and how that influences how we teach.

qualitative approaches to assessment in this type of assessment the student is asked to include written information to demonstrate their knowledge and understanding. They might complete an essay or reflective account. Qualitative feedback to the student might include comments on particular areas of their work such as *you make a good point about your experience of using reflective model X in an emergency situation compared with a routine situation.*

Quality Assurance Agency (QAA) works across all four nations of the UK. It is the independent body entrusted with monitoring and advising on standards and quality in UK higher education, The QAA sets and monitors the standards of UK higher education. This includes the UK Quality Code for Higher Education.

reasonable adjustments are measures put in places to ensure disabled students are enabled to achieve their full potential in both practice and campus-based learning environments. These may include altered shift patters or specialist equipment such as speech recognition software for students with dyslexia.

recognition of prior learning (RPL) a process used by AEIs that takes into account any previous learning undertaken by a student. This learning may have been formal learning carrying academic credit, such as a course. Or it may be less formal learning, for example someone who has undertaken an audit as part of their role. They can use this to evidence the necessary knowledge required for a module or course. RPL is often used as part of the entrance requirements for a course or to enable students to reduce the number of modules they need to study on a course.

self-efficacy is about our confidence in succeeding in a given situation or to perform a task.

summative assessment is usually completed at the end of a period of study, such as a module or placement. Students are graded on the performance either pass/fail or specific grade and this is used to determine their progression, final mark or grade or classification.

uni-professional working a single professional group, such as nursing or social work, often working in isolation to each other and with prescribed roles.

References

Aked, J, Marks, N, Cordon, C and Thompson, S (2008) *Five Ways to Wellbeing: A Report Presented to the Foresight Project on Communicating the Evidence Base for Improving People's Wellbeing.* London: New Economics Foundation. Available online at: https://neweconomics.org/uploads/files/8984c5089d5c2285ee_t4m6bhqq5.pdf

Aliakbari, F, Parvin, N, Heidari, M and Haghani, F (2015) Learning theories application in nursing education. *Journal of Education and Health Promotion,* 4. Available online at: www.ncbi.nlm.nih.gov/pmc/articles/PMC4355834

Allen, S (2010) The revolution of nursing pedagogy: a transformational process. *Teaching and Learning in Nursing,* 5(1): 33–38.

Anonymous (2013) How can staff sickness rates be reduced in the NHS? *Nursing Times,* 109(13): 11.

Arnold, EC and Boggs, KU (2015) *Interpersonal Relationships-E-Book: Professional Communication Skills for Nurses.* St Louis, MO: Elsevier Health Sciences.

Askew, S and Lodge, C (2000) Gifts, ping-pong and loops-linking feedback and learning. In Askew, S (ed) *Feedback for Learning.* London: Routledge.

Astrup, J (2018) The big story: raising standards for students. *Midwives Magazine.* Royal College of Midwives. Available online at: www.rcm.org.uk/news-views-and-analysis/news/the-big-story-raising-standards-for-students

Atkins, J (2002) Interprofessional education today, yesterday and tomorrow. *Learning in Health and Social Care,* 1(3): 172–76.

Atkinson, S and Williams, P (2011) The involvement of service users in nursing students' education. *Learning Disability Practice (through 2013),* 14(3): 18.

Austin, Z (2018) How to design and use learning objectives in clinical teaching. *Lung Cancer,* 15: 5.

Bandura, A (1977) *Social Learning Theory.* Englewood Cliffs, NJ: Prentice-Hall.

Boud, D (2015) Feedback: ensuring that it leads to enhanced learning. *The Clinical Teacher,* 12(1): 3–7.

Boud, D and Molloy, E (2013) Rethinking models of feedback for learning: the challenge of design. *Assessment & Evaluation in Higher Education,* 38(6): 698–712.

Boud, D, Cohen, R and Sampson, J (2014) *Peer Learning in Higher Education: Learning from and with Each Other.* Abingdon: Routledge.

Brooks, DC (2016) *ECAR Study of Undergraduate Students and Information Technology* (Vol. 4, No. 3, p2).

Burton, J and Jackson, N (eds) (2003) *Work-based Learning in Primary Care*. Abingdon: Radcliffe Publishing.

Caldwell, J, Dodd, K and Wilkes, C (2008) Developing a team mentoring model. *Nursing Standard*, 23(7): 35–39.

Carson-Stevens, A, Davies, MM, Jones, R, Chik, ADP, Robbé, IJ and Fiander, AN (2013) Framing patient consent for student involvement in pelvic examination: a dual model of autonomy. *Journal of Medical Ethics*, 39(11): 676–80.

Chandan, M and Watts, C (2012) Mentoring and pre-registration nurse education. Available online at: www.willriscommission.org.uk/__data/assets/pdf_file/0009/479934/Mentoring_and_preregistration_nurse_education.pdf

Chapman, A (2017) Using the assessment process to overcome imposter syndrome in mature students. *Journal of Further and Higher Education*, 41(2): 112–19.

Cheever, S and De Waal, A (2015) of Talion. *The Journal of Pastoral Care* 44(2) (Summer 1990): 131–37.

Christensen, M, Aubeeluck, A, Fergusson, D, Craft, J, Knight, J, Wirihana, L and Stupple, E (2016) Do student nurses experience imposter phenomenon? An international comparison of final year undergraduate nursing students' readiness for registration. *Journal of Advanced Nursing*, 72(11): 2784–93.

Chuan, OL and Barnett, T (2012) Student, tutor and staff nurse perceptions of the clinical learning environment. *Nurse Education in Practice*, 12(4): 192–97.

Clarke, D, Williamson, GR and Kane, A (2018) Could students' experiences of clinical placements be enhanced by implementing a Collaborative Learning in Practice (CliP) model? *Nurse Education in Practice*, March: 1–3.

Costello, J (1989) Learning from each other: peer teaching and learning in student nurse training. *Nurse Education Today*, 9(3): 203–206.

Cox, E, Bachkirova, T and Clutterbuck, DA (eds) (2014) *The Complete Handbook of Coaching*. London: Sage/Learning Matters.

Cummings, J and Bennett, V (2012) Compassion in practice. NHS Commissioning Board, Department of Health.

Davies, HT and Nutley, SM (2000) Developing learning organisations in the new NHS. *BMJ: British Medical Journal*, 320(7240): 998.

Dean, E (2012) Building resilience. *Nursing Standard (through 2013)*, 26(32): 16.

Department for Health and Human Services (2009) *Writing SMART Objectives*. Available online at: www.cdc.gov/healthyyouth/evaluation/pdf/brief3b.pdf

Disability Rights Commission (1985) *Maintaining Standards: Promoting Equality*. Available online at: http://dera.ioe.ac.uk/1985/1/maintaining_standards_formal_investigation_full_report.pdf

Duffy, K (2003) *Failing Students: A Qualitative Study of Factors that Influence the Decisions Regarding Assessment of Students' Competence in Practice.* Glasgow: Caledonian Nursing and Midwifery Research Centre.

Duffy, K (2013) Providing constructive feedback to students during mentoring. *Nursing Standard (through 2013)*, 27(31): 50.

Duffy, K (2015) Integrating the 6Cs of nursing into mentorship practice. *Nursing Standard (2014+)*, 29(50): 49.

Duffy, K and Hardicre, J (2007a) Supporting failing students in practice. 1: Assessment. *Nursing Times*, 103(47): 28–29.

Duffy, K and Hardicre, J (2007b) Supporting failing students in practice. 2: Management. *Nursing Times*, 103(48): 28–29.

Egan, G (2013) *The Skilled Helper: A Problem-management and Opportunity-development Approach to Helping.* Belmont, CA: Cengage Learning.

Eick, SA, Williamson, GR and Heath, V (2012) A systematic review of placement-related attrition in nurse education. *International Journal of Nursing Studies*, 49(10): 1299–1309.

Eller, LS, Lev, EL and Feurer, A (2014) Key components of an effective mentoring relationship: a qualitative study. *Nurse Education Today*, 34(5): 815–20.

Ellis, P and Bach, S (2015) *Leadership, Management and Team Working in Nursing.* London: Sage/Learning Matters.

English National Board for Nursing, Midwifery and Health Visiting (ENB) (2001) *Placements in Focus: Guidance for Education in Practice for Health Care Professions.* English National Board for Nursing, Midwifery and Health Visiting.

Evans, D and Brown, J (2017) Students in difficulty. In Cantillon, P, Wood, D and Yardley, S (eds) *ABC of Learning and Teaching in Medicine.* London: BMJ Books.

Fawcett, TJN and Rhynas, SJ (2014) Re-finding the 'human side' of human factors in nursing: helping student nurses to combine person-centred care with the rigours of patient safety. *Nurse Education Today*, 34(9): 1238–41.

Felstead, IS and Springett, K (2016) An exploration of role model influence on adult nursing students' professional development: a phenomenological research study. *Nurse Education Today*, 37: 66–70.

Francis, R (2013) *Report of the Mid Staffordshire NHS Foundation Trust Public Inquiry: Executive Summary (Vol. 947).* London: The Stationery Office. Available online at: http://webarchive. nationalarchives.gov.uk/20150407084231/http://www.midstaffspublicinquiry.com/ report

Gainsbury, S (2010) Nurse mentors still 'failing to fail' students. *Nursing Times*, 106(16): 2.

Gibbs, G (1988) *Learning by Doing: A Guide to Teaching and Learning Methods.* Further Education Unit.

Gravells, A (2017) *Principles and Practices of Teaching and Training: A Guide for Teachers and Trainers in the FE and Skills Sector.* London: Sage/Learning Matters.

Griffiths, L, Worth, P, Scullard, Z and Gilbert, D (2010) Supporting disabled students in practice: a tripartite approach. *Nurse Education in Practice*, 10(3): 132–37.

Glasper, A (2016) Moving from a blame culture to a learning culture in the NHS. *British Journal of Nursing*, 25(7): 410–11.

Hallin, K (2014) Nursing students at a university: a study about learning style preferences. *Nurse Education Today*, 34(12): 1443–49

Hamshire, C, Willgoss, TG and Wibberley, C (2012) 'The placement was probably the tipping point': the narratives of recently discontinued students. *Nurse Education in Practice*, 12(4): 182–86.

Haraldseid, C, Friberg, F and Aase, K (2016) How can students contribute? A qualitative study of active student involvement in development of technological learning material for clinical skills training. *BMC Nursing*, 15(1): 2.

Hart, PL, Brannan, JD and De Chesnay, M (2014) Resilience in nurses: an integrative review. *Journal of Nursing Management*, 22(6): 720–34.

Health and Safety Executive (no date) *Stress at Work*. Available online at: www.hse.gov.uk/stress/signs.htm

Health Education England (no date) *Comeback: Supporting Nurses to Return to Practice*. Available online at: https://comeback.hee.nhs.uk/

Health Education England (2015) *Managing Foundation Programme Doctors with Differing Needs*. Available online at: https://madeinheene.hee.nhs.uk/Portals/0/Policies/Foundation%20Specific/Managing%20FD%20different%20needs/Managing%20Foundation%20Programme%20Doctors%20with%20Differing%20Needs.pdf?ver=2016-05-31-134330-893

Health Education England (2016) *Values Based Recruitment Framework*. Available online at: https://www.hee.nhs.uk/our-work/values-based-recruitment

Health Education England (2017) *Multi-professional Framework for Advanced Clinical Practice in England*. Available online at: https://hee.nhs.uk/sites/default/files/documents/Multi-professional%20framework%20for%20advanced%20clinical%20practice%20in%20England.pdf

Hearle, D, Lawson, S and Morris, R (2016) *A Strategic Guide to Continuing Professional Development for Health and Care Professionals: The TRAMm Model*. Keswick, Cumbria: M&K Update Ltd.

Helminen, K, Tossavainen, K and Turunen, H (2014) Assessing clinical practice of student nurses: views of teachers, mentors and students. *Nurse Education Today*, 34(8): 1161–66.

Helminen, K, Coco, K, Johnson, M, Turunen, H and Tossavainen, K (2016) Summative assessment of clinical practice of student nurses: a review of the literature. *International Journal of Nursing Studies*, 53: 308–19.

HM Treasury (2015) *Spending Review and Autumn Statement 2015*. London: HM Treasury.

Honey, P and Mumford, A (2000) *The Learning Styles Helper's Guide.* Maidenhead: Peter Honey Publications.

Howatson-Jones, L (2016) *Reflective Practice in Nursing.* London: Sage/Learning Matters.

Hughes, LJ, Mitchell, M and Johnston, AN (2016) 'Failure to fail' in nursing: a catch phrase or a real issue? A systematic integrative literature review. *Nurse Education in Practice,* 20: 54–63.

Hunt, LA, McGee, P, Gutteridge, R and Hughes, M (2012) Assessment of student nurses in practice: a comparison of theoretical and practical assessment results in England. *Nurse Education Today,* 32(4): 351–55.

Hunt, LA, McGee, P, Gutteridge, R and Hughes, M (2016) Manipulating mentors' assessment decisions: do underperforming student nurses use coercive strategies to influence mentors' practical assessment decisions? *Nurse Education in Practice,* 20: 154–62.

Huybrecht, S, Loeckx, W, Quaeyhaegens, Y, De Tobel, D and Mistiaen, W (2011) Mentoring in nursing education: perceived characteristics of mentors and the consequences of mentorship. *Nurse Education Today,* 31(3): 274–78.

Jarrett, C (2010) Feeling like a fraud. *Psychologist,* 23(5): 380–83.

Jervis, A and Tilki, M (2011) Why are nurse mentors failing to fail student nurses who do not meet clinical performance standards? *British Journal of Nursing,* 20(9): 582–87.

Jones, K, Warren, A and Davies, A (2015) *Mind the Gap: Exploring the Needs of Early Career Nurses and Midwives in the Workplace.* Birmingham: Health Education England.

Kelton, MF (2014) Clinical coaching: an innovative role to improve marginal nursing students' clinical practice. *Nurse Education in Practice,* 14(6): 709–13.

Kemper, KJ, Mo, X and Khayat, R (2015) Are mindfulness and self-compassion associated with sleep and resilience in health professionals?. *The Journal of Alternative and Complementary Medicine,* 21(8): 496–503.

Keogh, B (2013) *Review into the Quality of Care and Treatment Provided by 14 Hospital Trusts in England: Overview Report. NHS England.* Available online at: www.nhs.uk/NHSEngland/bruce-keogh-review/Documents/outcomes/keogh-review-final-report.pdf

Kirkwood, TB, Bond, J, May, C, McKeith, I and Teh, MM (2014) Foresight Mental Capital and Wellbeing Project: Mental Capital Through Life: Future Challenges. *Wellbeing: A Complete Reference Guide,* pp1–90.

Koen, MP, Van Eeden, C and Wissing, MP (2011) The prevalence of resilience in a group of professional nurses. *Health SA Gesondheid (Online),* 16(1): 1–11. Available online at: https://hsag.co.za/index.php/hsag/article/view/576

Kramer, U (2010) Coping and defence mechanisms: what's the difference? – second act. *Psychology and Psychotherapy: Theory, Research and Practice,* 83(2): 207–21.

Lave, J and Wenger, E (1991) *Situated Learning: Legitimate Peripheral Participation.* Cambridge: Cambridge University Press.

Lawson, L (2010) *Supporting Mentors and Clinical Educators: A Collaborative Project into the Development of Knowledge and Skills to Enhance Clinical Education Practice.* University of Hertfordshire, unpublished report.

Lestander, Ö, Lehto, N and Engström, Å (2016) Nursing students' perceptions of learning after high fidelity simulation: effects of a three-step post-simulation reflection model. *Nurse Education Today,* 40: 219–24.

Lewin (2007) Clinical learning environments for student nurses: key indices from two studies compared over a 25 year period. *Nurse Education in Practice*, 7: 238–46.

Lobo, C, Arthur, A and Lattimer, V (2014) Collaborative Learning in Practice (CLiP) for pre-registration nursing students. Health Education England, University of East Anglia. Available online at: www.charleneloboconsulting.com/wp-content/uploads/CLiP-Paper-final-version-Sept-14.pdf

MacIntosh, T (2015) The link lecturer role: inconsistent and incongruent realities. *Nurse Education Today*, 35(3): e8–e13.

Martins, MC, Chaves, C and Campos, S (2014) Coping strategies of nurses in terminal ill. *Procedia-Social and Behavioral Sciences*, 113: 171–80.

McDermid, F, Peters, K, Daly, J and Jackson, D (2016) Developing resilience: stories from novice nurse academics. *Nurse Education Today*, 38: 29–35.

McDonald, S and Ahern, K (2002) Physical and emotional effects of whistle blowing. *Journal of Psychosocial Nursing and Mental Health Services*, 40(1): 14–27.

McDonough, K (2016) How to teach interprofessional learners. In Mookherjee, S and Cosgrove, E (eds) *Handbook of Clinical Teaching*. Switzerland: Springer.

McKellar, L and Graham, K (2017) A review of the literature to inform a best-practice clinical supervision model for midwifery students in Australia. *Nurse Education in Practice*, 24: 92–98.

Miller, L, Williams, J, Marvell, R and Tassinari, A (2015) *Assistant Practitioners in the NHS in England*. Skills for Health. Available online at: www.skillsforhealth.org.uk/images/resource-section/reports/Assistant%20Practitioners%20in%20England

National Nursing Research Unit (2009) Nursing competence: what are we assessing and how should it be measured? *Policy*. Issue 18. King's College London. Available online at: https://www.kcl.ac.uk/nursing/research/nnru/policy/Policy-Plus-Issues-by-Theme/Boundaries-regulation-competence/PolicyIssue18.pdf

Neenan, M and Dryden, W (2013) *Life Coaching: A Cognitive Behavioural Approach*. London: Routledge.

Newnham-Kanas, C, Morrow, D and Irwin, JD (2010) Motivational coaching: a functional juxtaposition of three methods for health behaviour change: motivational interviewing, coaching, and skilled helping. *International Journal of Evidence Based Coaching & Mentoring*, 8(2): 27–48.

NHS Choices (2017) *Moodzone: How to Deal with Stress*. Available online at: www.nhs.uk/conditions/stress-anxiety-depression/understanding-stress/

NHS Employers (2017) *Multigenerational Workforce*. Available online at: www.nhsemployers.org/your-workforce/plan/recruiting-from-your-community/engaging-with-and-recruiting-from-across-your-local-community/multigenerational-workforce

NHS England (2014) *Five Year Forward View*. Available online at: www.england.nhs.uk/wp-content/uploads/2014/10/5yfv-web.pdf

NHS England (2015) The NHS Constitution. *The NHS Belongs to Us All*. London: NHS England.

NHS Executive (2015) New 'duty of candour' guidance published for NHS staff. *Workforce and Training News*. Available online at: www.nationalhealthexecutive.com/Health-Care-News/new-duty-of-candour-guidance-published-for-nhs-staff

Nursing and Midwifery Council (no date) *Professional Duty of Candour Guidance.* Available online at: www.nmc.org.uk/standards/guidance/the-professional-duty-of-candour/read-the-professional-duty-of-candour/

Nursing and Midwifery Council (2008) *Standards to Support Learning and Assessment in Practice: NMC Standards for Mentors, Practice Teachers and Teachers.* London: Nursing and Midwifery Council.

Nursing and Midwifery Council (2010) *Standards for Pre-registration Nursing Education.* London: Nursing and Midwifery Council.

Nursing and Midwifery Council (2011) *Standards for Competence for Registered Midwives.* London: Nursing and Midwifery Council. Available online at: www.nmc.org.uk/globalassets/sitedocuments/standards/nmc-standards-for-competence-for-registered-midwives.pdf

Nursing and Midwifery Council (2015) *The Code: Professional Standards of Practice and Behaviour for Nurses and Midwives.* London: Nursing and Midwifery Council. Available online at: www.nmc.org.uk/globalassets/sitedocuments/nmc-publications/nmc-code.pdf

Nursing and Midwifery Council (2017a) *How to Revalidate with the NMC: Requirements for Renewing Your Registration.* Available online at: www.nmc.org.uk/globalassets/sitedocuments/revalidation/how-to-revalidate-booklet.pdf

Nursing and Midwifery Council (2017b) *Enabling Professionalism in Nursing and Midwifery Practice.* London: Nursing and Midwifery Council. Available online at: www.nmc.org.uk/globalassets/sitedocuments/other-publications/enabling-professionalism.pdf

Nursing and Midwifery Council (2017c) *Raising Concerns: Guidance for Nurses and Midwives.* London: Nursing and Midwifery Council.

Nursing and Midwifery Council (2018a) *Future Nurse: Standards of Proficiency for Registered Nurses.* London: Nursing and Midwifery Council. Available online at: www.nmc.org.uk/globalassets/sitedocuments/education-standards/future-nurse-proficiencies.pdf

Nursing and Midwifery Council (2018b) *Part 2: Standards for Student Supervision and Assessment.* London: Nursing and Midwifery Council. Available online at: www.nmc.org.uk/globalassets/sitedocuments/education-standards/student-supervision-assessment.pdf

Nursing and Midwifery Council (2018c) Meeting of the Council (March), Council Papers. Available online at: https://slidelegend.com/council-papers-march-2018-nmc_5ae35e147f8b9a18998b45a4.html

Nursing and Midwifery Council (2018d) *Standards Framework for Nursing and Midwifery Education. Part 1 of Realising Professionalism: Standards for Education and Training.* London: Nursing and Midwifery Council. Available online at: www.nmc.org.uk/standards-for-education-and-training/standards-framework-for-nursing-and-midwifery-education/

Olson, MH (2015) *Introduction to Theories of Learning.* New York: Routledge.

Palmer, S (2008) The PRACTICE model of coaching: towards a solution-focused approach. *Coaching Psychology International,* 1(1): 4–8.

Pålsson, Y, Mårtensson, G, Swenne, CL, Ädel, E and Engström, M (2017) A peer learning intervention for nursing students in clinical practice education: a quasi-experimental study. *Nurse Education* Today, 51: 81–87.

Pollock CHF, Rice AM and McMillan A (2015) Mentors' and students' perspectives on feedback in practice assessment: a literature review. *NHS Education for Scotland.* Available online at: www.nes.scot.nhs.uk/media/3288312/mentors_and_students_perspectives_on_feedback_in_practice_assessment.pdf

Powell, T (2009) *The Mental Health Handbook 3rd edition: A Cognitive Behavioural Approach.* London: Speechmark Publishing Ltd.

Pritchard, E and Gidman, J (2012) Effective mentoring in the community setting. *British Journal of Community Nursing*, 17(3): 119–24.

Robinson, S, Cornish, J, Driscoll, C, Knutton, S, Corben, V and Stevenson T (2012) *Sustaining and Managing the Delivery of Student Nurse Mentorship: Roles, Resources, Standards, And Debates.* Report for NHS London 'Readiness for Work' programme. National Nursing Research Unit, King's College London. Available online at: www.kcl.ac.uk/nursing/research/.../Nurse-Mentorship-Short-Report-Nov12.pdf

Rogers, CR (2004) *On Becoming a Person: A Therapist's View of Psychotherapy.* London: Constable.

Rosser, E (2017) Education does matter: nursing apprenticeships in the workforce. *British Journal of Nursing*, 26(7): 434.

Royal College of Nursing (no date) *Patient Safety and Human Factors.* Available online at: www.rcn.org.uk/clinical-topics/patient-safety-and-human-factors

Royal College of Nursing (2007) *Guidance for Mentors of Nursing Students and Midwives: An RCN Toolkit.* London: RCN.

Royal College of Nursing (2016a) *RCN Factsheet: Continuing Professional Development (CPD) for Nurses Working in the United Kingdom (UK).* Available online at: www.rcn.org.uk/about-us/policy-briefings/pol-1614

Royal College of Nursing (2016b) *RCN Mentorship Project 2015: From Today's Support in Practice to Tomorrow's Vision for Excellence. Rapid Evidence Review.* London: RCN. Available online at: www.rcn.org.uk/professional-development/publications/pub-005454

Royal College of Nursing (2017a) *Helping Students Get the Best from Their Practice Placements: A Royal College of Nursing Toolkit.* Available online at: file://staffhome.hallam.shu.ac.uk/STAFFHOME1/1/hscjl/MyWork/Jos%20stuff/send%20to%20Julie/PUB-006035.pdf

Royal College of Nursing (2017b) *Response to NMC Consultation Document on: Standards of Proficiency for Registered Nurses; Education Framework; Standards for Education and Training; Prescribing and Standards for Medicines Management.* Available online at: www.rcn.org.uk/-/media/royal-college-of-nursing/.../2017/.../pdf-006447.pdf

Royal College of Nursing (2017c) Reasonable adjustments: the peer support service guide for members affected by disability in the workplace. Available online at: www.rcn.org.uk/professional-development/publications/pub-006595

Scott, SV (2014) Practising what we preach: towards a student-centred definition of feedback. *Teaching in Higher Education*, 19(1): 49–57.

Seymour-Walsh, A (2016) Addressing clinician burnout: how can we build resilience in tomorrow's health professionals? *Resuscitation*, 106: e48–e49.

Shin, IS and Kim, JH (2013) The effect of problem-based learning in nursing education: a meta-analysis. *Advances in Health Sciences Education*, 18(5): 1103–20.

Sonnak, C and Towell, T (2001) The impostor phenomenon in British university students: relationships between self-esteem, mental health, parental rearing style and socioeconomic status. *Personality and Individual Differences*, 31(6): 863–74.

Steinert, Y (2008) Teaching rounds: the 'problem' junior: whose problem is it? *British Medical Journal*, 336(7636): 150.

Su, WM and Osisek, PJ (2011) The revised Bloom's Taxonomy: implications for educating nurses. *The Journal of Continuing Education in Nursing*, 42(7): 321–27.

Tasselli, S (2015) Social networks and inter-professional knowledge transfer: the case of healthcare professionals. *Organization Studies*, 36(7): 841–72.

Tee, SR, Owens, K, Plowright, S, Ramnath, P, Rourke, S, James, C and Bayliss, J (2010) Being reasonable: supporting disabled nursing students in practice. *Nurse Education in Practice*, 10(4): 216–21.

Tillett, R (2003) The patient within: psychopathology in the helping professions. *Advances in Psychiatric Treatment*, 9(4): 272–79.

Vinales, JJ (2015) Exploring failure to fail in pre-registration nursing. *British Journal of Nursing*, 24(5): 284–88.

Whitbourne, SK (2011) The essential guide to defence mechanisms, *Psychology Today*. Available online at: www.psychologytoday.com/gb/blog/fulfillment-any-age/201110/the-essential-guide-defense-mechanisms

Whitelock, D, Thorpe, M and Galley, R (2015) Student workload: a case study of its significance, evaluation and management at the Open University. *Distance Education*, 36(2): 161–76.

Williams, A (2013) The strategies used to deal with emotion work in student paramedic practice. *Nurse Education in Practice*, 13(3): 207–12.

Willingham, DT, Hughes, EM and Dobolyi, DG (2015) The scientific status of learning styles theories. *Teaching of Psychology*, 42(3): 266–71.

Willis Commission (2012) *Quality with Compassion: The Future of Nursing Education.* Available at: www.williscommission.org.uk/__data/assets/pdf_file/0007/495115/Willis_commission_ report_Jan_2013.pdf

Willis, P and Shape of Caring Review (2015) *Raising the Bar: Shape of Caring: A Review of the Future Education and Training of Registered Nurses and Care Assistants.* Health Education England.

World Health Organisation (2013) *Interprofessional Collaborative Practice in Primary Health Care: Nursing and Midwifery Perspectives Six Case Studies.* Available online at: www.who.int/hrh/resources/IPE_SixCaseStudies.pdf?ua=1

Zerach, G, Solomon, Z, Cohen, A and Ein-Dor, T (2013) PTSD, resilience and posttraumatic growth among ex-prisoners of war and combat veterans. *Israel Journal of Psychiatry and Related Sciences*, 50(2): 91–99.

Index